Hygiene and Morality

Lavinia L. Dock

Nabu Public Domain Reprints:

You are holding a reproduction of an original work published before 1923 that is in the public domain in the United States of America, and possibly other countries. You may freely copy and distribute this work as no entity (individual or corporate) has a copyright on the body of the work. This book may contain prior copyright references, and library stamps (as most of these works were scanned from library copies). These have been scanned and retained as part of the historical artifact.

This book may have occasional imperfections such as missing or blurred pages, poor pictures, errant marks, etc. that were either part of the original artifact, or were introduced by the scanning process. We believe this work is culturally important, and despite the imperfections, have elected to bring it back into print as part of our continuing commitment to the preservation of printed works worldwide. We appreciate your understanding of the imperfections in the preservation process, and hope you enjoy this valuable book.

By Lavinia L. Dock

A TEXT-BOOK OF MATERIA MEDICA FOR NURSES. Fourth Edition, Revised and Enlarged. Cr. 8vo. Net, $1.50

HISTORY OF NURSING. The Evolution of the Methods of Care for the Sick from the Earliest Times to the Foundation of the First English and American Training Schools for Nurses. By LAVINIA L. DOCK, R.N., and M. ADELAIDE NUTTING, R.N. Two volumes, 8vo. Fully illustrated. Net, $5.00.

Hygiene and Morality

A Manual for Nurses and Others, Giving an Outline of the Medical, Social, and Legal Aspects of the Venereal Diseases

By

Lavinia L. Dock, R.N.

Graduate of Bellevue Hospital Training School, Resident Member of the Nurses' Settlement, New York, Secretary of the International Council of Nurses

G. P. Putnam's Sons
New York and London
The Knickerbocker Press

Copyright, 1910
BY
LAVINIA L. DOCK

Published, June, 1910
Reprinted, October, 1910; February, 1911
January, 1912; April, 1912

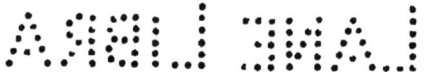

The Knickerbocker Press, New York

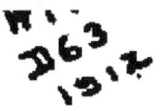

PREFACE

THE plan of this manual has grown from the scope of a paper presented by the author to the International Congress of Nurses in London, in July, 1909, in which the chief purpose aimed at was the same as has been here followed, namely, to reiterate the social significance of the venereal diseases and the crusade upon which women should enter in regard to them. Therefore, though the book is meant primarily for the nursing profession with its many thousands of members, it has not been arranged simply as a text-book on diseases, and the author hopes it may be useful to many other women as well. The author's thanks are to be cordially expressed to Dr. Elizabeth Hurdon and Dr. Florence Sabin, both of the Johns Hopkins Medical School, for reading the text on the Venereal Diseases; to Dr. Caroline Hedger, member of the Chicago Society of Social Hygiene, who has read the whole text; to Dr. Louis I. Dublin of Brooklyn for information relating to industrial insurance, and to Miss Alice Henry of Hull House for notes on maternal subsidies.

LAVINIA L. DOCK, R. N.

The Nurses' Settlement
265 Henry St., New York.

CONTENTS

CHAPTER		PAGE
	PART I.—THE VENEREAL DISEASES	1
I.	SYPHILIS	3
II.	GONORRHŒA AND CHANCROID	40
	PART II.—PROSTITUTION	57
I.	CONTROL AND REGULATION OF PROSTITUTION	59
II.	THE WHITE SLAVE TRAFFIC	104
	PART III. THE PREVENTION OF VENEREAL DISEASE	127
I.	UNDERLYING PRINCIPLES OF PREVENTION	129
	APPENDICES	171
	INDEX	195

Part I. The Venereal Diseases

CHAPTER I

SYPHILIS

THE venereal diseases are, in the commonly accepted order of their gravity: Syphilis; Gonorrhœa; Chancroid. The first mentioned is, by many modern medical writers, classed by itself, as will be explained later. For a long period in medical history, these three were all believed to be manifestations of one and the same disease. This confusion of ideas continued until the identification of the specific causative germs brought definite understanding and gave a sound basis to theory.

HISTORICAL OUTLINE. Venereal diseases are of great, probably of unknown antiquity. Some writers say that gonorrhœa has always existed. Syphilis appears to accompany certain stages of civilisation, as at least some barbarous tribes are and have been free from it. It is known that it has been introduced into certain ones of such tribes by white men. This has recently occurred with decimating results in the case of the tribe of Baganzas in Central Africa.

Some medical historians affirm that syphilis was unknown in Europe before the discovery of America and that it was carried thence into Europe, having presumably had its source in the ancient civilisations of Central America. Prominent authorities hold this view, while others, also prominent, maintain that it has existed for many more centuries in Europe but has been confused with leprosy. The controversy is one of no more than academic interest. What is historically certain is, that an epidemic of syphilis of frightful virulence raged in Europe at the end of the fifteenth century, constituting a veritable plague, and that it spread to all the countries and corners of the continent. Since then, it has been ever present in a less spectacular, sub-acute form as an endemic disease. Though now less noticeable, it is no less pestilential; perhaps indeed it is even more dangerous by reason of its concealment, as it is thus able to promote undiscovered that racial degeneration which has been pointed out as one of its chief activities.

CAUSE OF SYPHILIS. Syphilis is caused by a

micro-organism called the *Spirochæte pallida* of Schaudinn. This micro-organism, the specific and invariable cause of syphilis, has not long been known with certainty, though long before its actual demonstration medical specialists had suspected its existence. Metchnikoff records the work of Donné, a French microscopist, who, in 1837, tried to learn from his microscope the exact nature of the genito-urinary discharge in both men and women. But his efforts resulted in nothing definite. In his day the germ theory was non-existent. After the work of Pasteur had given a new direction to medical and surgical study and had caused the doctrine of the action of micro-organisms as the cause of infectious disease to be accepted, active search and research went on in laboratories all over the world, to discover the germs of this as well as of other diseases. But for twenty years or more the definite attempts made by Weigart, Lustgarten, Metchnikoff, and many others to find the cause of syphilis ended in failure. Finally a commission of experts was formed under the lead of Schulze, Professor of Zoölogy in the University of Berlin, and the investigation directed toward the discovery of the syphilitic virus was by him entrusted to Schaudinn and Hoffman, who, finally, were successful in their search, and in 1905 were able to demonstrate the micro-organism which is now generally accepted by the medical profession as the cause of syphilis.

SCHAUDINN'S DISCOVERY. It was shown that two varieties of *Spirilla* were to be found in normal and in diseased states of the genital organs. The first variety, called *Spirilla refringens*, may be existent in either state, and may be demonstrated in different pathological conditions, both non-syphilitic and syphilitic in character. The second variety, the *Spirilla pallida*, is only found in syphilis, not even in other venereal diseases unless syphilis is also present.

THE SPIROCHÆTE PALLIDA. The *Spirochæte pallida* is classed among the *Spirilla*. It is not yet definitely settled whether it belongs to the bacteria or the protozoa. This uncertainty, which is practically unimportant, may be ended any day, as active study of its nature is constantly going on under such masters as Metchnikoff, Roux, and others. Bloch, a high authority, calls it a protozoön.

Metchnikoff points out the fact that the female genital organs are the home of other forms of *Spirilla*, which may at times be mistaken for the *Spirochæte pallida*. Beside the *Spirochæte refringens* there is still another, the *Spirochæte balanitis*, and these, being sometimes found in lesions of syphilis, have been called secondary organisms.

The *Spirochæte pallida* is a delicate organism. It is smaller and slenderer than the other *Spirilla* mentioned, and has more spirils. It has been called "*pallida*," the pale *Spirochæte*, because of the technical difficulty of staining it for observation in laboratory work. Schaudinn, it is said, first named it *Spirochæte pallida*, later called it *Spirochæte pallidum*, and still later *Treponema pallidum*. The first name remains the one in general use.

It only survives for a few hours—six, Andrews says—outside of the human body. After that its infectious power is lost. It is destroyed by heating for an hour to 51 degrees Centigrade (124° Fahr. approximately). It needs moisture, and if dried dies quickly, but even with moisture present it is very perishable when removed from its human host. This readily perishable quality and early loss of pathogenic power is of the highest importance in considering the subject of contagion by direct mechanical contact with infected objects, as will be seen later, and has a definite bearing on practical methods of disinfection and on the avoidance of direct infection from inanimate objects and personal contact.

So far, efforts to cultivate the *Spirochæte* in artificial media have not succeeded, but this, too, may be accomplished any day, as all the famous bacteriological laboratories of the world are experimenting on this line.

GENERAL RESULTS OF EXPERIMENTS. Experimental work so far has been successful in demonstrating the *Spirochæte pallida* in the primary, secondary, and tertiary lesions of syphilis; in the lymphatic organs and the lymph; in the saliva and urine; in arterial lesions; in the fœtus, and in the newborn congenitally syphilitic infant, which, indeed, always shows enormous numbers of the specific germ in its various organs.[1] It has also been occasionally demonstrated in the blood. Further, experimental work, chiefly that carried on in the Pasteur Institute under the

[1] Metchnikoff.

direction of Metchnikoff, and by Neisser in Java, has been successful in transmitting the disease syphilis to certain varieties of apes, and in thus clearing up some important and formerly unknown facts and principles that are of value for early and correct diagnosis and treatment.

Thus it has been shown that the virus of syphilis can be demonstrated in the internal organs within sixteen days after infection, and long before the usual time of appearance of the earliest outward sign of the disease, namely, the "primary sore."[1] Unremitting attempts made to obtain a prophylactic serum or mitigated virus such as has been successfully produced for diphtheria, tetanus, etc., have so far been only partially successful, but, though some scientists regard the production of such a serum or vaccine as a doubtful possibility, the efforts to produce it will no doubt go on until it has been accomplished.

The proof of the early extinction of the life of the germ after being removed from the body is one of the important results of experiment, and, in the work with apes, a number of data, valuable for diagnosis and treatment, have been secured, notably that of the "serum diagnosis" of Neisser,

[1] Neisser.

Wassermann, and Brink. This is based upon the natural reaction that takes place in the blood after the introduction of certain poisons, and the appearance in the blood of so-called "antibodies," or natural antagonists to the poison in question. These "antibodies," normally not demonstrable by ordinary methods of examination, may increase and be found in large quantities under the stimulus of the disease poison. Their presence in syphilis is now regarded as an important passive aid to diagnosis, though their absence would not necessarily prove the non-existence of the disease.

The effects of the drugs used in the clinical treatment of syphilis, especially mercury, have also been extensively and usefully studied in the course of animal experimentation.

SYMPTOMS AND COURSE OF SYPHILIS. Syphilis has been defined as a specific disease of slow evolution, propagated by inoculation (acquired syphilis), or by hereditary transmission (congenital syphilis).[1]

Acquired syphilis is invariably due to direct contact with the discharges or secretions of a patient already suffering from the disease. It is

[1] Osler.

supposed that some minute break or abrasion in the skin or mucous membrane exposed to the virus is a condition of infection, though this break may be too minute to be noticeable. The squamous epithelium seems to be the primary channel of infection. The germ of syphilis cannot be transmitted through the atmosphere in dust particles, as may happen in the case of the tubercle bacillus.

Syphilis is an infectious fever, running a slow or chronic course, and, like other fevers, it has a period of incubation followed by acute symptoms including skin eruptions and general disturbances of the health, and it has, later, sequelæ or remote consequences of definite and varied, often of frightful character. Unlike other fevers, which run their course in a few weeks, this one lasts for months and even for years, while its sequels, like those of scarlet fever, are permanent and terrible in their nature.

The course of syphilis is divided into three stages: primary, secondary, and tertiary.

PRIMARY STAGE. The primary stage begins with the close of the incubation period, while incubation itself may take from ten days to seven weeks after the time of exposure to infection. This variance in time is supposed to be due to the varying number of *Spirochæte pallida* present in the infectious material or discharges by which the disease is carried. The average period of incubation is three or four weeks. During this time there are no signs of disturbance, and the abrasion through which the poison has been received, heals.

Finally, at the end of the incubation period, a small red papule appears at the point of inoculation. It may or may not enlarge. A little later it breaks down in the centre, forming an ulcer, small or large as the case may be, but, as a rule, single. This is known as the "hard chancre," from the fact that the tissues about it are indurated and dense, with a gristle-like feeling, and it is known as the "primary lesion" or "initial sore" of syphilis. The discharge from this ulcer is highly contagious, yet, if the ulcer is of small size, it may be readily overlooked. In the primary stage there may be no disturbance of the general health, nor any symptoms that attract attention. The primary stage continues for from one to three months with no other signs of trouble than the primary lesion itself. This quiescent period is sometimes called the second incubation period.

At its close, rarely later than the twelfth week, an active set of constitutional symptoms come on.

SECONDARY STAGE. The poison has now been distributed by the lymphatic system, as evidenced by enlargement of the glands in all parts of the body. There may be fever, more or less marked and of variable character, and skin eruptions, also of very varied characteristics, the most usual being a rash resembling measles which appears first on the chest and abdomen, spreading thence to other parts of the body. One form of the eruption resembles smallpox; others bear resemblance to skin diseases of different origin and varying features. There is severe nocturnal headache and pain in the bones, with a general feeling of illness. The inner surfaces of the mouth and all the structures of the pharynx and throat may become sore, red, and swollen, sometimes so acutely so that solid food cannot be swallowed. The mucous patches which are among the most significant and special symptoms of syphilis may appear on all or any parts of the inner surfaces of the mouth and gums, tongue, tonsils, and pharynx. They may also appear at the corners of the lips, or in the nasal lining, or in the folds of the axillæ and the perineum, or even between the toes. The mucous patch is a flat, greyish ulcer, which secretes a copious, virulently infectious discharge. Other symptoms of the secondary stage are syphilitic iritis, inflammation of the periosteum and of the joints, alopecia, syphilitic onychia, and condylomata, or the "syphilitic warts" which are frequently found in the vulvar region. The labyrinth of the ear may be involved and deafness result.

TERTIARY STAGE. The oncoming of the tertiary stage cannot always be separated from the secondary stage by a definite line, nor can the symptoms of the secondary and tertiary periods always be distinctly separated in classification, as, in some cases, symptoms usually regarded as late ones may appear early, or, again, the stages may not run a perfectly typical course. Nor does the tertiary stage always develop. Tertiary symptoms, like sequels of other contagions, are not wholly inevitable. They may be averted by early, careful treatment carried on for a sufficient length of time.

When the third stage of syphilis does occur, its onset may not take place for months or even years after the primary sore. During a long period the patient may have believed himself to be entirely well and free from danger. This slowness of development and insidious latency of the disease constitutes one of its most dread features. Andrews says: "No other communicable disease continues its manifestations after twenty and even fifty years after the original infection."

It is believed that the chief cause contributory to the development of tertiary symptoms is inadequate treatment in the very early stages. As a result of this inadequacy of care it may happen that cases which appeared mild and insignificant at the outset, and which, in consequence, may have received only brief or superficial treatment, develop most malignant and violent tertiary symptoms. There are, however, some cases where the virulence of the poison defies all, even early, treatment.

As a rule, the general condition of the patient and of his surroundings have much bearing upon the probable results of treatment. If the general health is good, surroundings sanitary, and treatment adequate and faithfully followed, the patient may generally feel hopeful of cure.

Alcoholism makes the prognosis much worse, and bad hygienic living conditions also add to a discouraging outlook. The parasites may not be actually killed, but only rendered latent and may, in consequence, produce tertiary symptoms at a remote period.

The typical characteristics of the third period of syphilis are "gummata" or soft tumors which may develop in any set of tissues, from the hard bony structure through the whole range of internal organs to the brain and skin. These tumors or gumma tend to ulceration and destruction of tissues, and produce the deformities sometimes seen, such as the destruction of the bridge of the nose, etc. Skin eruptions of a more formidable type than the earlier ones, and having a more pronounced tendency to ulcerate, appear in this stage.

CONGENITAL SYMPTOMS. Every feature of the acquired disease except the primary sore, says Dr. Osler, may be seen in the congenital form. The baby born with syphilis is wasted and withered, with the wrinkled "old" looking little face; fissures at the corners of the mouth; a discharge from the nostrils, "snuffles"; ulcerated lips; excoriated buttocks; dry and unhealthy skin; eruptions, especially about the extremities:

some or all of these symptoms may be present. The baby with these marked evidences of disease is not likely to live. Or, the baby may be born healthy looking and well, but after a few weeks' time may develop snuffles, eruptions, fissures about the mouth, loss of hair and eyebrows, or other less markedly characteristic symptoms. This process usually occurs between the third and twelfth week. Children with congenital syphilis, says Osler, rarely thrive. Certain ones may improve or recover, but there is apt to be a return of the disease at puberty. Even those who recover from the early symptoms do not develop normally. They often have a wizened, wasted look, their growth is slower, and there is a frequent condition known as "infantilism" which gives, for instance, to the youth of nineteen the appearance of a boy of twelve.

About the time of puberty, the child with inherited syphilis may develop persistent eye and ear diseases. Of all the organs of special sense, the eye is the one most frequently attacked. Disease of bones may appear early or late, and the late case of hereditary syphilis may display the dread gummata and end in general paresis. The lesions of the third stage are also infectious, though, as they are often situated in deep seated tissues, there is less opportunity for the infection to be conveyed to others.

The congenitally syphilitic infant is intensely infectious. Fournier says: "Nothing is so dangerous to its surroundings as a syphilitic infant."

SYPHILIS HEREDITARY IN THE LITERAL SENSE. Syphilis is hereditary, not in the sense of an inherited predisposition only, as is the case with tuberculosis (once believed to descend as an actual entity from one generation to another), but the disease itself may be inherited. In other words, the new-born baby may come into the world with the *Spirochæte pallida* present in enormous numbers in all or in any of its tissues. Morrow says: "Syphilis is the only disease which is transmitted in full virulence to the offspring."

HEREDITY TO THE THIRD GENERATION. It is a matter of some difference of opinion and controversy whether syphilis is transmissible to the third generation. The French school, fairly generally, some American writers, and Hutchinson, the English authority, take the negative, while many others withhold a positive pronouncement. In the absence of a definite certainty, however, one cannot but recall the words of the Old Testament, "The sins of the fathers are visited upon the children, even unto the third and fourth generations," and surmise that they may reflect the accumulated wisdom of ages of experience. In this connection it may be remembered too that the exact study of syphilis is now, according to distinguished medical writers, only in its infancy.

It is supposed that, in a large number of cases, the syphilitic taint is derived from the father only; that the semen conveys the *Spirochæte pallida* directly to the product of conception. It is also authoritatively taught that, if the mother alone has transmitted the disease to the offspring the danger is graver—the fatality to the children more overwhelming than if the father alone has transmitted it. Recent studies emphasise the predominant part of the mother in heredity.

A phenomenon first pointed out by a noted surgeon of Dublin, Colles, and named after him, is that of a mother who, herself apparently free from the disease, gives birth to a child showing congenital taint, and can herself nurse her baby without becoming infected by it, whilst the most healthy wet-nurse nursing the same baby becomes infected. But it seems to be a question whether this mother, who appears to be immune, really is so or not. Osler speaks of her as receiving a "protective inoculation." Hutchinson makes the observation that it would be important to know how many such mothers showed tertiary symptoms in later life. This is at present not known, but he believes there is proof that there are many, and holds this to be corroborative of the view that such mothers really do receive an infection during pregnancy. The whole subject is one of present incertitude, and with further research is likely to be completely revised. Another phenomenon which has been called after Profeta is that of a child apparently healthy which nurses its syphilitic mother without becoming infected. This also must be taken with reserve as needing further exact investigation.

Finally, it is supposed that the offspring may escape infection altogether if the mother is not infected until late in pregnancy, especially if not until after the seventh month.

IMMUNITY. A study of the most recent writings gives the impression that it is regarded as, on the whole, doubtful whether a true natural immunity against syphilis exists in the human individual. D'Arcy Power says that, as far as is now known, no healthy person is proof against syphilis, but that any one who is directly exposed to it, in the literal sense of having the *Spirochæte pallida* introduced into the lymphatic system, will contract the disease. Nor is there a certainty as to acquired immunity. Neisser holds that, in the case of syphilis, there is no such thing as the acquired immunity which is familiar as following upon some other contagious diseases—that is, when an individual, having once had a contagious disease and having been cured, is thereafter insusceptible to it. He teaches, as the result of his investigations with animals, that cases which appear to display immunity and resistance to fresh infection are really not cured, but have the *Spirochæte pallida* still present in their tissues, and that cases which had been really cured by treatment, *i. e.*, when the microscope proved that the *Spirochæte* had actually been killed, were susceptible to new infection.

While it is not always correct to make precise deductions from animal experimentation for man he believes that this is also true of human beings—that cases of so-called "immunity" are not such, but that these individuals still have the *Spirochæte pallida* present in their tissues. In October, 1908, he stated that no method of procuring active or passive immunity, nor mode of treatment with immunising substances, had been discovered.

On this point, Hutchinson says that he has seen seven cases of true second attacks of syphilis at intervals of from eighteen months to twelve years after the first attack. The possibility of a second attack, is therefore, he believes, only the expression of the efficiency of the treatment of the first. Lang of Vienna says that for a long time there was a belief in the absolute immunity conferred by a first attack of syphilis but that this belief was disproved by Zeissl and others. Reinfection, he holds, can only occur in individuals who have been perfectly cured. Those in whom the disease is still present are not susceptible to new infection.

Reinfected cases usually run a mild course. So, too, it is believed that races in which syphilis has long been widely prevalent show a less obvious type of symptom.

RELATION OF SYPHILIS TO THE NERVOUS SYS-

TEM. The relation of syphilis to a number of the disorders of the nervous system had only been imperfectly understood up to the time of the discovery of the *Spirochæte pallida*. Careful studies are now being pressed along this line, and it cannot be doubted that the rapid progress of modern medical science will continuously throw new light upon these obscure problems, to the incalculable benefit of the human race.

Some diseases of the nervous system are directly due to syphilis, as hemiplegia from syphilitic degeneration of the walls of arteries; and paralysis or convulsions due to syphilitic tumors of the brain or those lying at the roots of nerves.

Again, some of the most formidable nervous diseases, classed as para-syphilitic, are regarded not as in themselves syphilitic, but as resulting in some way from the virus of syphilis or from the changes it has brought about in the organs. Prominent among these are locomotor ataxia and the general paralysis of the insane. It was formerly held that the first mentioned disease might arise from other causes; that, though the great majority of cases were of definitely syphilitic origin, a certain percentage of the remainder must not be so regarded. But the more recent writers tend to the assumption that the syphilitic taint is invariably to be found in the previous history, even though it may be many years, or a full generation, earlier.[1]

THE RELATION OF SYPHILIS TO CARCINOMA. Recent writers point out the great importance of further investigation into the obscure relationship between syphilis and carcinoma. D'Arcy Power states that cancer is peculiarly liable to occur in the tissue which has undergone a chronic syphilitic inflammatory process, and speaks of the virus of syphilis as "preparing the tissues" for cancer, especially that form of it known as epithelioma. While there is no reason for supposing that syphilis is closely related to carcinoma yet its importance as a predisposing or favourable condition for the development of this terrible affliction should give added weight to every argument for the extirpation of syphilis from human society.

SYPHILIS AND TUBERCULOSIS. The author just quoted points out the inter-relation between syphilis and tuberculosis, and believes that

[1] Mott in *British Medical Journal*, Feb. 27, 1909.

syphilitic tissues are more liable to infection by the bacillus of tuberculosis than other equally ill-nourished tissues are, if syphilis-free. He emphasises the interaction between the two diseases, while, at a recent meeting of the American Society of Sanitary and Moral Prophylaxis the statement was made that, if syphilis could be wiped out, a vast amount of the tuberculosis now existent would also disappear.

SYPHILIS AND OTHER DISEASES. In a general way it may be stated that syphilis constitutes a predisposition to bear all other constitutional diseases badly. The intemperate, the tuberculous, the rheumatic, the malarial patient all suffer more, and find themselves in a less hopeful condition when syphilis or the syphilitic degeneration is present as a complication.

SYPHILIS AND ALCOHOLISM. A relationship or affinity appears to exist between syphilis, alcohol, and prostitution which unites them in a trio of great and evil menace to health. Dr. Morrow says:

Instruction would be incomplete without a warning as to the influence of alcohol in the instigation of immoral relations and as one of the most powerful auxiliaries of sexual contamination. The rôle of alcohol in the propagation of venereal diseases has not been sufficiently appreciated, and the consideration that every repressive measure against alcohol will be an important prophylactic measure against the spread of venereal diseases has not received the attention it deserves. Perhaps more than any other agency, alcohol relaxes the moral sense while it stimulates the sexual impulse.

Neisser speaks of "the fatal rôle of alcoholism which drives innumerable young men to exaggerated exercise of the sexual functions"; and Pontoppidan says:

Alcohol is an inducing and even a downright cause of the rise and propagation of venereal diseases. Alcohol paralyses the will and understanding, and stimulates sexual and sentimental emotion. Abstinence and temperance movements must be taken as important allies in the prevention of venereal diseases.

Medical statistics show that an excessive proportion of venereal disease has been contracted while under the influence of alcohol. Dr. Forel's investigations suggest an affinity between syphilis and tissues that are habituated to alcohol. He finds that alcohol is oftener the exciting cause of infection in men than in women, while it oftener induces women to commit the first irregular act. Dr. Morrow states also that chronic alcoholism is a powerful factor in bringing on the development of severe and extensive lesions of the skin and mucous membranes; that it promotes the cerebral disorders of syphilis, and causes the disease to run into the third stage.

Loxton emphasises the necessity of cutting off alcohol entirely in the treatment of all venereal diseases, and cites cases of gonorrhœa where abrupt relapses with acute symptoms followed immediately after alcoholic drinks had been taken.[1]

Ravogli says:

Alcoholism when associated with syphilis is also a most important factor in crime. We know the deleterious influence of alcohol in individuals affected with syphilis,—so much so that the French speak of a special kind of syphilis, *la syphilis alcoholisée.* Some writers indeed go so far as to claim that the general paralyses of tertiary syphilis only occur in those who have been addicted to drink.

SYPHILIS AND CRIME. A suggestive article by Ravogli on syphilis in relation to crime gives the scientific reasons of the author for believing

[1] *British Medical Journal*, Feb. 27, 1909.

that the injurious action of the syphilitic virus upon the vascular system and the structures of nerves is an explanation of much of the degeneracy that is evidenced by crime, and especially by cruel and persecutory kinds of crime where the perpetrator enjoys the sufferings of others. He quotes Barthélemy, who says that "the great class of heredo-syphilitics forms the ranks of the degenerate, unbalanced, obnubilated mattoids," and that this heredity, with alcoholism, is the most effective cause of human degradation. Ravogli says: "The existence of moral insanity admits of no doubt, and that it is often the result of syphilitic alterations of blood-vessels is easy to demonstrate."

While he does not mean to be understood as saying that syphilis is the determining cause of crime, he does believe that it is one of the predisposing factors of crime, and he then goes on to say:

A strange relation exists between syphilis, crime, and prostitution—cases of prostitution which cannot be explained by poverty or by special accident have to be attributed to hereditary syphilis. Prostitution and crime go hand in hand, and in the families where the brothers are criminals the sisters are prostitutes. Syphilis is the tie between crime and prostitution when it causes the affections of the nervous system resulting in moral degeneration.

STATISTICAL ESTIMATES OF SYPHILIS. No comprehensive or general system of counting the cases of syphilis or the other venereal disorders is yet officially established in any country. The available statistics, therefore, being those collected by medical specialists in their own practice and in hospital records, though authoritative, and sufficiently startling, have not the extent of those collected by public bureaus or health departments. Nevertheless there are data enough to enable medical experts to make very definite assertions as to the prevalence of venereal diseases and their share in morbidity and mortality.

The general prevalence of syphilis is estimated at from five to eighteen per cent. of populations, some countries having a worse record than others. It is stated in medical writings that from ten to fifteen per cent. of the male population of Europe have syphilis.

Destruction of the foetus and a heavy infant mortality are prominent results of syphilis. Morrow says: "No disease has such a murderous influence upon the offspring." It is known that syphilis is responsible for a large percentage of all miscarriages, while the death-rate of congenitally syphilitic infants is described by the expression "Poly-Mortality."

Figures taken from European hospital records and from physicians' note-books, all classes of the community being considered as one, show a double fatality when both parents are infected, or an infant death-rate of sixty-eight per cent. In private practice only, the social status here being rather superior, the infant mortality is sixty or sixty-one per cent. Free public hospitals, where the most indigent cases find refuge, show the worst figures, from eighty-four to eighty-six deaths in every hundred infants. One in every four or five lives long enough to pass the heritage on. Physicians record instances of the extinction of entire families from syphilis. Fournier cites one such case, where, to 157 births, there were 157 deaths from this cause. In the *Transactions* of the American Society of Sanitary and Moral Prophylaxis the statement is made that in France alone syphilis kills twenty thousand children annually. The ages at which syphilis is, in a large proportion of cases, contracted, give melancholy testimony to the prevalent neglect of the young. There are authentic medical figures showing that from thirty to forty per cent. of the cases of this disease are infected between the ages of fourteen and twenty years.

Besides the hereditary infection of children by their parents the infection of wives by their husbands is common. Morrow's records show that, of all the women suffering from syphilis who attended the clinics of a large hospital, seventy per cent. were respectable married women who had been infected by their husbands. He says further that "possibly ten per cent. of men who marry infect their wives with venereal disease," and his estimation of the total number of syphilitics in the United States is two million.

It is believed that, generally speaking, about ten per cent. of all cases of syphilis are transmitted accidentally in various ways like ordinary contagions, that is to say, not by sexual contact. Thus, of 887 cases of syphilis in women, recorded by Fournier, 842 had been acquired in sexual contact, while the others had been accidentally conveyed by ordinary contact, through instruments, tubes, utensils, etc., or by caring for or suckling diseased infants, etc.

THE SOURCE AND SPREAD OF SYPHILIS. A distinction must be made between (a) cause; (b) source or breeding-place; (c) mode of spread of any infectious disease.

The cause of every such disease is a special micro-organism. The sources or breeding-places where these organisms flourish and congregate vary, as we know, while the means by which they are disseminated broadcast also vary, almost to infinity.

Those contagions that are called, familiarly, filth diseases, do not cease being filth diseases when they are conveyed into clean homes to strike down cleanly living individuals. In the study of every infectious disease knowledge of the breeding-place or native haunt of its germ is of the utmost importance for practical hygiene. Thus the world has rung with the announcements of the mosquito carriers of yellow fever and malaria and with the exploits of those medical heroes who sacrificed their lives in the search for this knowledge;—again, in the case of tuberculosis, information as to the breeding-places and modes of dissemination of the tubercle bacillus is published in public places, told in public lectures, and, indeed, almost cried in the streets.

In the case of typhoid fever, it is accepted by all intelligent people as a civic crime to neglect water supplies. So in the case of every infectious germ; as its habitat and ways of spreading are learned, the knowledge is given freely and fully to the world. In the case of syphilis, and of other venereal diseases as well, though their specific micro-organisms have not long been identified, their breeding-places and most prominent mode of transmission have been well known for many years by the medical and legal professions and by sophisticated members of the laity, but, because of the perplexing, complicated, and difficult social web in which they were woven, these facts have been concealed and an absolutely opposite policy has prevailed from that followed, for instance, with tuberculosis. With the latter, full publicity: with the former, until most recently, almost unbroken secrecy. Every one talks of tuberculosis; almost no one of venereal disease. It is true that tuberculosis also was not made a matter of public, national importance until its curable, preventable, and non-inheritable nature was discovered. This gives hope for believing that venereal diseases also may be brought into the open, since it can be shown that they are not only curable, but, more than any others, preventable, since their prevention may be a matter of choice and of the individual will. To these hopeful facts the certainty of the relentless hereditary transmission of syphilis should act as a powerful spur.

BREEDING-PLACE OF SYPHILIS AND THE VENEREAL DISEASES. The breeding-place of all venereal diseases without exception is in the social institution called prostitution, or sexual promiscuity: in the debasement and degradation of what should be the highest and most revered of physical powers, those involved in the act of generation. Bred and cultivated in prostitution, venereal diseases spread thence through the community, attacking the innocent as well as the guilty, the pure as well as the impure, just as typhoid fever is no respecter of persons, no matter how strict their own personal sanitary standards may be.

How, or why, the parasitic powers of the *Spirochæte pallida* first declared themselves in unlawful, not in lawful sexual intercourse, is a mystery. But it is certain that this organism is never met with in the relation of marriage unless it has been brought from without. Excesses in the marriage relation, though productive of other evils, do not bring on venereal diseases. If, as some writers state, even polygamy does not promote them, then it would seem as if the original exciting cause favourable to the parasitic vigour of the *Spirochæte pallida* must have been in some way related to the numbers and variety of male beings who practised a heterogeneous promiscuity. Howsoever their derivation might be traced, prostitution is now as certainly the abiding-place and inexhaustible source of this as of other germs of venereal disease, as the marshy swamp is the abode of the malaria-carrying mosquito, or the polluted water supply of the typhoid bacillus. Pontoppidan of Copenhagen says: "Even if contagion is carried in different ways, its origin can nearly always be traced back to prostitution." And Bulkley says: "Prostitution undoubtedly stands foremost as a cause of syphilis and far outweighs all other causes together." Again, he says: "In the enormous majority of cases syphilis is acquired in illicit intercourse." Osler says, "Inextricably blended with it [the social evil] is the prevention of syphilis." Morrow speaks of "The original source of these infections in that irregular commerce between the sexes known as prostitution."

Since the discovery of the germ of syphilis there appears some tendency on the part of some medical writers to remove syphilis from the list of venereal diseases. As has been mentioned, it is frequently classified separately, thus: "Syphilis and the Venereal Diseases." The argument is that, with the fuller knowledge of its many modes of transmission, its constitutional features, and hereditability, its venereal stigma should be removed. Yet, as, although a germ disease, its germ does not appear to be distributed generally, like the pus-producing germs; as the disease syphilis never breaks out afresh under normal conditions, nor develops from the germ in the course of moral living, but is cultivated in morally unclean sexual relations, then it does not seem incorrect to call it a venereal disease, even though it may be communicated to moral and innocent individuals in non-venereal ways arising in the ordinary contact of daily life. The important things to know are: That it is cultivated in prostitution and thence spread through the community in ways which are to be mentioned in detail. These ways are classified by Bulkley as follows:

I. Inherited. II. Marital. III. Extra-genital.

I. The hereditary communicability of syphilis has been discussed.

II. The marital mode of transmission is the infection of one partner (usually the wife) by the other during the performance of the act of generation. As this act offers the most favourable possible opportunity for infection of such a nature to be carried, it results that by far the greatest proportion of cases that are innocently or accidentally received—a proportion that is variably estimated—have been conveyed in the marriage relation.

III. With the knowledge of the micro-organism and its presence in all syphilitic lesions and in the discharges from primary sores, ulcers, mucous patches, secretions of the mouth and nose, etc., it may be readily understood that the opportunities for infection to be conveyed in the ordinary processes of daily life, especially when people live under crowded or uncleanly conditions, are very numerous.

That syphilis is not more frequently conveyed by incidental contact than is actually the case is due to the, fortunately, very short life of the germ outside the human body.

All of the common acts of daily life may serve as means of infection during the brief period of the parasite's existence, viz., eating and drinking from cups and saucers, knives, forks, and spoons that may have been in contact with the lips of a syphilitic; putting pencils, pins, money, whistles, or any other article in the mouth after it may possibly have been in that of an infected person.

Towels, handkerchiefs, pillow-cases, or any article of bedding as well as water-closet seats and bath-tubs may serve as carriers. Surgical and dental instruments, shaving apparatus, medical appliances in familiar use, as bulbs, sprays, douche bags, spatulas, and syringes, may convey the poison. Cases have been recorded where it has been inoculated during the process of vaccination, and occasional known instances of this kind have had much to do with strengthening the objections of anti-vaccinationists and intensifying the popular prejudice against vaccination that is found in some communities. Syphilis has also been conveyed in circumcision and other slight operations.

Laundresses and rag-pickers have not infrequently been infected by soiled or cast-off clothing;

physicians and surgeons are always liable to this danger in the course of their professional work; midwives are exposed during the delivery and care of patients; nurses have been infected while caring for patients, the nature of whose illness had not been made known to them, and with whom they were therefore not as vigilantly on guard as they should have been.

Most dangerous of all the avenues of accidental infection is contact with the person of the syphilitic, on account of the probability of then receiving germs that are living and virulent. Any such contact with the lips, teeth, or tongue is especially dangerous, such as kissing (an act which is known to have been the cause of many innocent cases), playful biting or mouthing (such as is often carried on playfully between children and adults), sucking wounds, licking with the tongue, etc.

The syphilitic baby is an especially infectious object because of the many necessities of the baby for close personal care and handling in feeding and bathing it.

CHAPTER II

GONORRHŒA AND CHANCROID

GONORRHŒA; ITS SPECIFIC MICRO-ORGANISM. Gonorrhœa is caused by an organism called *Gonococcus gonorrhœæ* which was discovered by Neisser in 1879 and has been especially studied and described by Bumm. As it is usually seen in pairs, it is also called the *Diplococcus gonorrhœæ* or the *Micrococcus* of Neisser. It is cultivable with difficulty, and does not survive many transplantations, yet transplanting does not lessen its virulence. It is always found in gonorrhœal pus, but is never found in other inflammatory conditions unless these are of gonorrhœal origin. It is said to perish quickly in sunlight and to be killed in a few hours by drying. Experimentation with it in the inoculation of animals has been attended with special and unusual difficulties.

The *Gonococcus gonorrhœæ* can live for years, or indefinitely, in the human tissues in a dormant or latent state, latent gonorrhœa being frequent in both men and women. This characteristic, unknown until the day of bacteriological study with the microscope, and not immediately discovered even then, gives the disease a specially uncertain character and makes it quite as treacherous as syphilis, if not even more so.

After remaining latent for a long time, perhaps for years, the organism of gonorrhœa, if conveyed to the sound and healthy tissues of another individual (such tissues being spoken of, in regard to the organism, as "virgin," or "sterile" tissues), finds its most favourable conditions for growth and then excites an actively acute inflammation and displays its utmost virulence.

HISTORY OF GONORRHŒA. Gonorrhœa is primarily a genito-urinary disease, and was formerly believed to be a purely local affection. It is supposed to be as old as the human race, and, like syphilis, its main line of propagation has always been in the promiscuous intercourse of prostitution, whence it has been disseminated in every direction. Ancient writings specify its symptoms with enough exactitude to make its identity plain. This identity was lost in the epidemic of syphilis in the 15th century, to which allusion has been made. During the 18th century the difference between syphilis and gonorrhœa might have been rediscovered, had not an inexact experiment of the celebrated John Hunter caused the medical profession to regard all venereal diseases as one up to the time of the work of Ricord.

If syphilis has only been fairly well understood for the last half-century, gonorrhœa, at least in so far as women are concerned, has only been estimated according to its real gravity in the last decade, though Neisser made his discovery in 1879. In 1857 two medical writers, Bernitz and Goupil, had made studies of gonorrhœal infection of the Fallopian tubes, but had found no followers. In 1878 Noeggerath sounded a warning, declaring that individuals with gonorrhœa could remain infectious during a lifetime, but he was regarded as an alarmist and his statistics of the frequency of gonorrhœa in married men as exaggerations. Gonorrhœa had been regarded as an ordinary "catarrhal" inflammation of the mucous membrane, locating itself usually in the urethra, and as, in men, the disease was well known to be acquired in promiscuous sex relations, it was commonly regarded with indifference, or even with levity, as a proof of rakishness, the purulent discharge being colloquially described in military countries as the "goutte militaire."

In the light of modern knowledge of the disastrous part taken by the *gonococcus* of gonorrhœa in that sad array of obscure and unnecessary ailments which have been erroneously called "Diseases of Women," the traces of this levity make painful reading, found, as they are, even in medical writings of a generation ago or less. To-day, instead of being regarded as a local disease, gonorrhœa also, like syphilis, is known to develop constitutional disturbances of a serious and chronic nature, and suggestions are not wanting that the former point of view will soon be antiquated.

COURSE AND SYMPTOMS OF GONORRHŒA. Osler divides the course of gonorrhœa into three stages:

1. Primary infection.
2. Extension through the entire genito-urinary tract.
3. Systemic infection.

PRIMARY INFECTION. The period of infection is from twelve hours to a week or more, the average being one or two days. In adults the urethra is usually the point of infection, or, in women, it may be also the cervix uteri, for the reason that the delicate linings of these parts are only weakly resistant and are easily penetrated by the bacillus. The uninjured squamous epithelium of the adult is not easily infected. With little girls, infection usually attacks the vulva and vagina, by reason of their delicate structure in childhood.

The symptoms of the primary stage are those of an ordinary acute local infection, with itching and burning of the parts, redness and swelling, pains, often intense, on urination, and a discharge, first mucous and finally purulent, with œdema of the surrounding tissues, excoriations, multiple abscesses, and perhaps hemorrhage from swollen papillæ. To the eye there is nothing to distinguish the symptoms from those of an ordinary inflammation, and only the microscope makes the diagnosis positive. Formerly, it was believed that cure had taken place when the discharge ceased. It is now known that this is far from being the case.

SECOND STAGE. The inflammation now goes on and involves the organs of generation and the urinary tract, ascending the ureters and spreading, it may be, to the kidneys, where it may produce a fatal pyelitis. In women a large proportion of all cases of cystitis, salpingitis, metritis, ovaritis, and pelvic peritonitis, as well as many cases of infection after childbirth are caused by the *gonococcus*.

The most serious, because irreparable, action of gonorrhœa upon the organs of generation is to cause sterility in both men and women. The frequency with which this sequel occurs will be referred to under "Statistics." In women this sterility is sometimes brought about by occlusion or blocking of the Fallopian tubes. Again, there is what is called "one-child sterility." When this happens, the *gonococcus*, at first restricted in its location to the cervix uteri, is enabled owing to the relaxation of the parts after childbirth, to extend to the tubes and ovaries. Or, again, the necessity of complete operative removal of all the female organs of generation effectually puts an end to all expectations of maternity.

THE DESTRUCTION OF EYESIGHT. Calamitous as are the sequels of gonorrhœa to the adult, especially to the married woman, no other single effect wrought by it can compare with the tragedy of infants, blinded at birth by virulent gonorrhœal poison, which enters the eyes during the infant's passage through the vaginal canal. This, too, will be referred to under "Statistics." Gonorrhœal poison is most actively destructive of the cornea, and the danger of incurring blindness from having the eyes infected with pus or discharge containing this virus is equally as great for adults as for infants. The opportunity for infection is less, yet blindness of older children and adults from the *gonococcus* received from towels, sheets and pillow-cases, fingers, handkerchiefs, etc., is frequent, and cases have occurred where nurses have lost one or both eyes through lack of sufficient precautions.

THIRD STAGE. The constitutional forms of gonorrhœa include, besides disease of the kidneys already mentioned, gonorrhœal arthritis, an intractable and obstinate form of rheumatism, prone to relapses, and gonorrhœal endocarditis. These are regarded as its two most serious constitutional sequels. There is also a gonorrhœal septicæmia. Authorities mention a urogenital tuberculosis, to which chronic urethritis has the relation of a predisposing cause. Morrow speaks of this as a recent acquisition of knowledge, and adds that modern investigations are showing that it is possible for the *gonococcus* to be taken up by the blood and lymph and carried to all organs of the body, and that it may affect them all injuriously. It has been found in the brain and cord, the pleura, the liver, spleen, and kidneys, the endocardium, the sheaths of tendons and of joints, and in the periosteum. Finally, it may not be amiss to place under the constitutional effects of the *gonococcus* that innumerable army of chronically semi-invalided married women of all ages, who, without having clearly defined loss of health, "have never been well since married," whose whole existence is a drag and who have often failed to find the commiseration due them, this having indeed been oftener given to the husbands, whose lot in having ailing wives was all unknowingly due, in many cases, to their own transmission to these unsuspecting and unfortunate women of the deadly *gonococcus* of Neisser.

MODES OF TRANSMISSION. Though in the majority of cases the germ is conveyed during the act of coitus, it is also possible for it to be carried in the contact of daily life, and it is only the brevity of its existence after being dried that saves many cases from infection. Infection from unclean water-closet seats is frequent, instances having been known where a whole series of cases of vulvo-vaginitis have arisen from this cause. It is pointed out by medical writers that it is not necessary to conclude that little girls with a gonorrhœal discharge have been violated or addicted to bad practices (though such may have been the case) as it is quite possible for them to have contracted the disease from badly kept school closets, or from sleeping in the same bed and being contaminated by the sheets or clothing of diseased persons. Family towels under such circumstances are sources of danger, and public baths and tubs are also known to have been media of contagion.

IMMUNITY AND ANTI-SERUM TREATMENT. It is not believed that there is immunity against the *gonococcus*. Serum treatment has been tried in certain forms of constitutional disease, and beneficial results have been claimed in the case of rheumatism. The Lister Institute prepares an "Anti-gonococcus Vaccine," which is a preparation of dead *gonococci* that is said to be poisonous to the living germ.[1] It is probably too early to find anything quite authoritative upon this line of study.

The statistics of gonorrhœa are so startling as to seem almost incredible. Like those of syphilis, they are drawn from the records of hospitals and medical practitioners, as health boards ignore the existence of venereal diseases.

PREVALENCE OF GONORRHŒA. Morrow quotes Neisser to the effect that gonorrhœa is the most widespread and universal of diseases in the adult male. European records indicate that about seventy-five per cent. of all men have gonorrhœa.

Assuming that a somewhat better moral standard prevails in the United States, it is given as a conservative estimate that the prevalence of both gonorrhœa and syphilis among men is at least sixty per cent. Morrow says that it is impossible to estimate accurately the extent to which gonorrhœa is conveyed to wives in marriage, but that it is generally agreed that this is greater than is generally suspected. Statistics gathered in New York City by the Committee of Seven indicated

[1] *British Medical Journal*, Feb. 27, 1909.

that nearly thirty per cent. of all venereal diseases of women in that city had been transmitted in marriage by the husbands. The remainder (leaving out hereditary transmission and accidental infection) would probably be found among prostitutes. As to these unfortunate centres of infection, J. Taber Johnson estimates, conservatively, that at least thirty per cent. of their whole mortality is due to gonorrhœa.

STERILITY. Neisser regards gonorrhœa as responsible for more than forty-five per cent. of sterile marriages, while Morrow points out that these figures refer to primary, not to secondary sterility, which is additional. Gonorrhœa is the foremost cause of male sterility. One specialist found thirty cases of male sterility in ninety-six sterile marriages, while the statement is made by Morrow that men are ultimately responsible for from fifty to seventy-five per cent. of all sterility in married life. In from twenty to twenty-five per cent. of such cases, the husband is sterile. In the others, he has infected the wife, making her sterile.

The extent of secondary sterility is not known. A major share, then, of all sterility is to be laid at the door of the *gonococcus*.

DISEASES OF WOMEN. The responsibility of the *gonococcus* in causing these diseases is variably estimated by different surgeons, ranging from forty to eighty per cent. All cases of pus in the Fallopian tubes are gonorrhœal, while at least fifty per cent. of all gynæcological operations are necessita ed by the *gonococcus*. This is a conservative estimate, some gynæcologists giving figures from their own practice that are much higher.

BLINDNESS. Eighty per cent. of all the purulent ophthalmia of infants is gonorrhœal, and from fifteen to twenty-five per cent. of all the blindness in America is due to the same cause. Neisser says that Germany alone has 30,000 blind persons whose affliction was caused by gonorrhœal pus, while in Paris the institutions for the blind show that forty-five per cent. of the cases have been due to this infection.

SUMMARY OF SYPHILIS AND GONORRHŒA. The consensus of expert medical opinion is, that, as a depopulating factor, gonorrhœa is more formidable than syphilis, and that it is also more perilous to the wife. Syphilis is more destructive to the life of offspring; gonorrhœa more destructive to the female organs of generation and to the general health. The hereditary quality and slow development of syphilis constitute its chief terrors, but the treacherous nature and persistent vitality of the *gonococcus* make gonorrhœa almost, if not quite, as terrible. Syphilis is, as a rule, more curable. The prognosis of gonorrhœa is always most uncertain. Both show certain types which are believed to be incurable.

Taking them together, they seem to exhibit the true race suicide, and both, says Taber Johnson, are intimately connected with the degeneration of races and the downfall of nations. Grandin says: "Man, largely through ignorance of the calamities following the misuse of this [the reproductive] instinct, has converted it into one for the extermination of the species."

CHANCROID (VENEREAL SORE; SOFT CHANCRE). The identity of the specific micro-organism of this last of the venereal diseases is still uncertain. A strepto-bacillus called the bacillus of Ducrey has been demonstrated in the soft chancre but it has not been proved to be its sole or specific cause.

Clinically, Bassereau, in 1856, determined that chancroid and syphilis were not the same. Nevertheless mistakes in confusing the two were frequently made until the organism of syphilis was discovered.

Venereal sore is by far the simplest and least dangerous of the three diseases under consideration. If treated promptly it is readily curable, though, if neglected, serious complications may ensue and cure be a more difficult matter. The incubation period is short; from several hours to several days. The first manifestation is a small nodule which proceeds rapidly toward suppuration, forming a painful ulcer with an intensely infectious discharge. The ulcer is deep and irregular, and its tendency is to spread and become multiple. Herein lies the danger of complications. Neglected ulcers may involve the glands and other parts in their vicinity with much consequent destruction of tissues locally, but the disease has no constitutional complications, nor has it sequels or belated manifestations. If properly treated from the outset, from four to six weeks suffice for cure. It only runs a prolonged course when neglected.

Venereal sore is always located on the genitalia.

SOURCES OF MATERIAL USED IN THE PREPARATION OF PART I

Bloch, Ivan, Der Ursprung der Syphilis. Jena, 1901.

Bolduan, Charles Frederick, M.D., Immune Sera (Appendix A: Serum Diagnosis of Syphilis). New York, 1908.

Bulkley, L. D., M.D., Syphilis in the Innocent. New York, 1894.

Bull, Ophthalmia Neonatorum and its Prophylaxis. In New York Medical Journal, May 15, 1909.

Findlay, Palmer, M.D., Gonorrhœa in Women. 1908.

Forel, August, M.D., Alcohol and Questions of Sex. In Report of the International Congress against Alcohol. 1905.

Forel, August, M.D., Alkohol und venerische Krankheiten. In Report of the International Congress against Alcohol, 1901.

Fournier, Alfred, Syphilis et Mariage. Paris, 1890.

Fournier, Alfred, Traité de la Syphilis. 1903.

Francke, Hermann, M.D., Beitrag zur Entwickelung bösartiger Geschwülste auf dem Boden alter Syphilitischer Narben. Würzburg, 1894.

Horaud, Réné Denis, M.D., Syphilis et Cancer. Lyon, 1907.

Johnson, J. Taber, M.D., The Influence of Gonorrhœa as a Factor in Depopulation. In Journal of the American Medical Association, August 10, 1907.

Metchnikoff, Élie, The Microbiology of Syphilis. In A System of Syphilis. Edited by D'Arcy Power and J. Keogh Murphy. London, 1908.

Morrow, Prince A., M.D., Gonorrhœæ Insontium, especially in Relation to Marriage. In New York Medical Journal, June 27 and July 4, 1903.

Morrow, Prince A., M.D., Prognosis and Relation of Syphilis

Sources of Material Used

to Marriage and Heredity. In Medical News, Sept. 2, 1907.

Morrow, Prince A., M.D., Social Diseases and Marriage. New York, 1905.

Mott, Syphilis. In British Medical Journal, Feb. 27, 1909.

Noeggerath, Emil, M.D., Die latente Gonorrhöe im weiblichen Geschlecht. Tr. Amer. Gyn. Soc. I. 1876.

Osler, William, M.D., Practice of Medicine. [Syphilis and Gonorrhœa.] London and New York, 1909.

Pontoppidan, Erik, M.D., What Venereal Diseases Mean and How to Prevent Them. Translated by W. Jessen.

Ravogli, Syphilis in Relation to Crime. In Ohio State Medical Journal, August, 1906.

Rogers and Torrey, The Treatment of Gonorrhœal Infection by a Specific Antitoxin. In Journal of the American Medical Association, Sept. 14, 1907.

System of Medicine, A. [Syphilis, etc.] Edited by Allbutt. London, 1906.

System of Syphilis, A. [Several Authors.] Edited by D'Arcy Power and J. Keogh Murphy. London, 1906.

Taylor, Prognosis in Syphilis. In Medical News, Sept. 2, 1907.

Torrey, An Antigonococcus Serum. In Journal of the American Medical Association, Jan. 27, 1906.

Part II. Prostitution

CHAPTER I

CONTROL AND REGULATION OF PROSTITUTION

THERE is a long and revolting history of the spasmodic attempts made from time to time during the past ages to control or punish prostitution. These attempts usually took the form of grotesque and brutal punishments for women, rarely for men. As a rule, the vicious male seems to have been overlooked or regarded as an insignificant factor in the problem. Punishments meted out to the woman were chiefly hypocritical or vindictive, not in the least preventive. Sometimes she was put into an iron cage and dipped into the river,—almost but not quite drowned; sometimes her nose was cut off; or she was whipped or compelled to wear a distinguishing dress. She has always been the victim of blackmail, and the methods by which this has been levied show a remarkable similarity right down through the ages to modern times: they were usually the enactment of non-preventive legislation, of a petty and harassing character, with the imposition of heavy fines for breach of observance. As such legislation simply made it more difficult for her to earn her bread in the only way open to her, it of course had to be violated, and the fines collected were divided between the accuser and the city government. Perhaps this mode of profit-sharing is not yet obsolete. It is needless to give much time to the painful details of centuries that are gone, and it will suffice to state simply that all such legislation rested, as it still does, on the acceptance (once unquestioned, but to-day no longer so) of the double standard of morals.

THE DOUBLE MORAL STANDARD. The essential feature of the double code or standard of morals is the entire absence of logical sequence. Therefrom results the injustice which is so striking, both from the standpoint of reason and of humanity.

The double standard tacitly permits men to indulge freely and unchecked in sexual irregularity without consequent loss of social standing, but it dooms the women who are necessarily involved in these irregularities to social ostracism and even to complete degradation.

In order to justify immoral practices among themselves and to have a plausible explanation ready if criticism offered, the doctrine of "physical necessity" has been invented for men by themselves, and has even been fortified by the positive teachings of prominent medical men. This doctrine, however, has never been extended to women, but, instead, the cowardly and cruel theory of innate depravity has been industriously disseminated as applying to "fallen women," thus skilfully ensuring an isolated position for these unfortunates, and effectually checking the outgrowth of pity for them among women of the protected classes. The practical results of this psychological jugglery have been, that, of two partners in one and the same act, neither one of whom could execute this act alone, and with whom, if the element of compulsion entered as a complication, it could not possibly be present in the case of the stronger partner,—men, the stronger, have remained free from blame; women, the weaker, have lived under a curse.

The fact that this way of regarding the woman concerned disproves the argument of "physical necessity" is only a part of the illogicality of the whole. It is evident that, if unregulated sexual practice were really necessary for men, there could be no element of shame or wrong in it, and there could therefore, obviously, be none for the women, for no act that is physically necessary is wrong, no matter how primal it may be.

In order to give strength to the social structure of prostitution, certain catch phrases have been passed current to act as mental hypnotics. For instance: "Prostitution must always exist, because it always has existed. Because it always has existed, therefore it always must exist." But it will be seen that, in company with this dictum, there have always gone very definite social and legal contrivances for ensuring its existence.

MODERN SYSTEMS OF REGULATION. In spite of the hitherto generally accepted belief in the necessity and right of men to practise sexual irregularity, the presence of prostitution in the community, though the inevitable result of such practice, has been regarded as a "social evil," partly because of its accompaniment of disease. In order to minimise the danger of disease while maintaining prostitution, associations of men have, in the past, set themselves to the task of making vice safe, by establishing systems of "Regulation" with medical inspection of female prostitutes. This device originated, it is said, with Napoleon Bonaparte, who thought it proper that women should be sacrificed to his soldiers, but did not wish the soldiers to be invalided. Since his day, regulatory systems have been established in most European countries. They vary somewhat in detail, and have been roughly divided into three types: the Scandinavian, the simplest and the most free from obnoxious features, combining a certain amount of police supervision with the compulsory reporting of venereal diseases and ample free medical service without a stigma attached to it; the German, sometimes called Neisser's system, highly complicated, with some slight attempt at more logic than is found in the third, called the unilateral system, and which has been adopted in many foreign countries, having reached its most notorious development in France, where, in the main, it is still in force, though it is probable that its downfall is near.

Opposed alike to all systems of state or police regulation of prostitution are the principles of the abolitionists, to be discussed later, and of the most modern and wisest socio-medical teachers.

The organisation of the unilateral system was as follows: A special department of police, called Morals Police (*Police des Mœurs*), was authorised to regulate and control prostitution as, in general, the head of the department saw fit; that is, ordinarily no public legislation defined their powers, but these were defined in police codes and in municipal ordinances. At the very outset, therefore, the women thus dealt with were excluded from the realm of the common law. The police had full power to arrest any women whom they might "believe" or "suspect," or "have reason to think" were immoral. This part of their powers rested chiefly upon a spy system of plain-clothes men, and anonymous letters were regarded as valuable sources of information. Arrest was followed by forcible medical examination, and the woman's name and address were inscribed on the lists in the police department. Every two weeks, or at other specified times, she was compelled to appear for examination, and, if found diseased, was confined in what was essentially a hospital prison.

The one-time head of the Morals Police of

Paris, when asked wherein lay the chief strength of his system, replied: "Arrests; always arrests; more and more arrests; that is our only hope."

That innocent women were often subjected to arrest and even imprisonment under this system was regarded as an unavoidable incident.

The unfortunates under police surveillance could never hope to escape from their life. Hounded by the police wherever they went, their outlook was described by Dr. Mireur, a defender of the system, in these words:

Cut off, not only from society but from heaven; from hope, and from the power to repent; nevertheless [he added] inscription and licensing are essential, indispensable, even as prostitution itself.

All systems of regulation alike brought into existence the licensed or "tolerated" houses of ill-fame, and such houses were protected by the police. Their keepers possessed a certain status by reason of this connection, and the appearance of recognition and support by the government confused the moral sense of the people. The keepers of such places have always been active supporters of regulative acts, because the women are then more completely helpless. A German chief of police admitted in his reports that the inscription of prostitutes by the police aggravated their abject condition in a horrible manner, while a member of the Reichstag once said: "It is well known that these are marked women and can never reform."

Such is the system, which, with varying modifications and with some differences of detail as to the harshness with which it has been or is enforced, still prevails widely under the general term, "The Continental System of the Regulation of Vice." It has recently been discarded in Italy, and has been strongly condemned by public commissions in France. Switzerland has given it up, except in Geneva, where it is in force in full ignominy.

It seems almost incredible that there are many who would willingly see this system implanted in the United States. More than one attempt has been made to introduce it into this country, and arguments in its favour are not infrequently heard. It is for this reason, among others, that women should be informed and alert upon a subject which would otherwise seem too horrible to contemplate.

The continental system of licensed houses of

ill-fame, as will be seen in a later chapter, has been the breeder for the white slave traffic, and these houses have been the main market of the traders and have afforded the trade its security. The unfortunate women hate the licensed houses because of their tyrannous features, and it has never been easy to fill the vacancies caused by disease and death. An organised system of supply and demand has therefore grown up, having developed early in the 19th century, not very long after the establishment of the regulation system. It must be explained that no government has ever consciously encouraged a white slave trade, but this has been the logical though unforeseen result of giving the tolerated houses a recognised status.

THE INTRODUCTION OF STATE REGULATION INTO GREAT BRITAIN. The strongest bulwark of regulated vice in all countries has been the military element. It has been a generally accepted understanding that armies of men must have free access to abandoned women, and it has always been a subject of serious concern with authorities to make this vice as safe as possible, in order that the fighting strength of regiments might be maintained in its efficiency. The necessary sacrifice of women involved in this point of view brought forth no protests, even from women, until the women of England were aroused to it by an attempt made to force the continental system upon that country.

THE CONTAGIOUS DISEASES ACTS. Early in the 19th century the military hierarchy had been desirous of establishing a regulated system in England, but the time did not seem propitious until well along in the mid-century, when the purpose crystallised.

A woman sounded the first warning. Harriet Martineau, with her finger always on the political pulse, foresaw the coming danger, and wrote several powerful letters of protest to the *Daily News* in 1859. In 1860 a Committee of the House of Lords sat to consider the advisability of introducing compulsory acts into India. Miss Martineau, in her autobiography, says that Florence Nightingale was called to give her opinion, and spoke strongly, with positive testimony against it. Nevertheless, between 1864 and 1869, the system was established in Great Britain by a series of Acts of Parliament passed with such haste and secrecy that, as is authoritatively stated in many published sources of reference, only about one tenth of the members knew of them. Introduced in late night sessions and rushed through with surreptitious haste, the first and second were only entering wedges, but the third established the full programme of regulation for all garrison towns and within a radius of fifteen miles around each one.

The first to give publicity to the new legislation, which was enforced with great secrecy, was the head of a Home for Girls, Daniel Cooper, who first suspected the onset of something new and menacing, and finally succeeded in obtaining a copy of the Acts. He exposed their iniquity, and was supported by two physicians, Dr. Charles Bell Taylor and Dr. Worth, who denounced them vigorously. But no headway was made in opposing them until all the moral forces of England were finally united under the leadership of Mrs. Josephine E. Butler,—one of the rare characters of the world, a perfect example of the exalted and fearless type of ideal womanhood;—one whose maternal protectiveness extended to every young and helpless creature.

SCOPE OF THE ACTS. The Acts empowered policemen in plain clothes, acting as spies, to arrest any woman in the territory covered by the law. The police were only obliged to "declare" that they "had reason for believing" the women to be immoral; it was therefore impossible to punish them for arresting innocent women, nor could informers be punished. Women thus arrested were requested to sign a paper called a "voluntary submission" (and ignorant ones were easily coerced into it) promising to present themselves at the periods ordered for medical examination, and, as an alternative, they had to defend their reputations in court. If they refused to submit to the medical examination, they could be sent to prison for disobedience. If, when examined, they were found to be diseased, they were committed to a hospital prison for compulsory treatment. If resistant, they were taken there by the police, and if they left it before being discharged they were liable to imprisonment with hard labour for one or two months. Under such a law, as an English writer pointed out, the police spies, acting on hints given them by persons acting in jealousy or revenge, or from motives of blackmail, "held the honour and reputation of every woman among the poorer classes absolutely at their disposal."

MRS. BUTLER'S CRUSADE. The women of England, united under Mrs. Butler's leadership in a national association, issued a declaration that the law was an insult and an outrage to every woman in the land, and protested against it on the following grounds: That laws are bound to define offences punishable by law. (No definition of prostitution was given in the Acts. It is indeed most difficult to define it technically and legally, and this difficulty has given rise to active controversy in every country where regulation has been in force.) That it was unjust to punish women only, and that the forced medical examinations were degrading punishments. That the Acts made it easier for young men to be impure. That the measures of enforcement were brutalising to all who took part in them. That venereal diseases had never been extirpated by such means, because their causes were moral and must be met by moral prevention. That to examine, treat, and isolate women only, while allowing infected men to go free, was a farce.

But a still higher ground was taken. Mrs. Butler insisted, in her speeches and writings, that the abolition movement was not merely a sex revolt, but was based on the conviction that impurity was as perilous for men as for women. It was as citizens first, and as women secondly, that they were in conflict with legislation that practically created a slave class. In her book, *The Constitution Violated*, Mrs. Butler defined clearly the

LEGAL AND CIVIC WRONGS OF REGULATION.

I. The first principle of jurisprudence in enlightened countries is that a suspected or accused person is protected against self-incrimination. The "voluntary submission" is a self-incrimination.

II. Enlightened countries hold an accused person innocent until he is proven guilty and so declared by a jury, but under the Contagious Diseases Acts the woman was held guilty until she could prove her innocence.

III. Constitutional law forbids indecent assault upon the person. The compulsory medical examination constituted an indecent assault.

Mrs. Butler showed further that the spy system necessitated by these laws subjected women to the arbitrary power of the police and removed them from the protection of the common law, and she made plain the inevitable confusion of the public conscience arising from the scruples of those persons who believe that the only wrong thing is disobedience to police regulations.

The protest embodying these civic and moral declarations is a historic human document which will be looked back upon with more and more veneration as the centuries pass. It was the first formal declaration of the revolt of women against the slavery of prostitution. It appeared in the *Daily News* on New Year's day, 1870, and was signed by two hundred and fifty of the great moral leaders among Englishwomen. Beginning with Harriet Martineau, there are many names known to literature, social reform, and advanced movements, and all the active suffragists of that day are enrolled there. Half-way down the column appears the name of Florence Nightingale.

THE STRUGGLE AGAINST THE ACTS. A long, desperate, and unremitting struggle followed the women's protest. Of three hundred prominent men in all walks of life, secular and religious, to whom, as an initial measure, Mrs. Butler first wrote letters of appeal for moral support, scarcely half a dozen gave a word of encouragement. Some declined to consider the subject, but most of them were silent. Mrs. Butler then turned for help to the public, and wrote her "Appeal to the People" in 1870. Tens of thousands of the working classes and plain people came to her support. Theirs were the daughters who were chiefly endangered.

Perhaps no other one woman has been more vilified or more venomously assailed by all the corrupt forces of society than was she. In several instances she narrowly escaped death from mob violence.

The contest was carried on for thirteen years, and the abolition party grew to a membership of 50,000, but during all this time political parties, even that with the great Mr. Gladstone at its head, resisted all appeals and ignored or belittled all testimony making for repeal of the Acts.

PROGRESS OF THE CRUSADE. In 1871, a Royal Commission recommended abolishing the compulsory examination, and raising the legal age of protection for girls from twelve years (as it then was) to fourteen. The first recommendation was not enacted into law until 1883. The second received some attention. The age of protection for little girls was with difficulty raised to thirteen, but not until 1885 was it possible to raise it to sixteen, so tenacious and determined was the resistance made to this amendment by the law-makers of the nation. As late as 1880, two members of Parliament spoke on the floor of the House in favour of reducing the age of protection for little girls to below twelve years.

In 1880, '81, and '82, a Select Committee was appointed to inquire into the whole question of the workings of the Acts, and a number of women were called to testify. Among them was Mrs. Butler, whose evidence was very full, drawn entirely from personal knowledge, and couched in language of great, often exalted beauty; of moving and stirring power.

This Committee, in its report, endorsed the Acts, but did not recommend their extension, and it was felt that this was a victory. In 1881, and '82, there was also a Select Committee of the House of Lords on the white slave traffic, and in 1885 the *Pall Mall Gazette* published revelations of so shocking a nature regarding the trade that Parliament, until then most reluctant to act, was driven to pass some protective legislation. The odious Acts were repealed. They still, however, continue in force as to some of their main features in distant subjected provinces of the Empire under the guise of "rules."

RALLY OF THE REGULATIONISTS. During the progress of the women's crusade the upholders of regulation in all countries had been gathering re-enforcements and trying to strengthen their position. Government officials, military authorities, and even physicians reasserted the right of men to enslave and destroy women for their sensual pleasure. The *Lancet* upheld the registration of prostitutes. At an International Medical Congress in Vienna in 1873, strong resolutions were passed urging a convention of all nations and international agreements to establish the compulsory system of supervision of women in all the great seaport cities of the world.

On that occasion one member present said: "*From the moment when prostitution shall become a regular and recognised institution, admitted and regulated by the state, its perfect organisation will become possible.*" Another made an even more astounding proposition based upon the inoculation theory. Resolutions were framed calling upon England to summon a congress to form an international league for the regulation of prostitution. Rev. C. S. Collingwood, an English clergyman, protested nobly against this proposition, and Mrs. Butler and her allies, alarmed by the rising tide of domination of the regulationists, determined to organise an international movement in opposition to them. Mrs. Butler therefore undertook a continental tour in 1874, the year of the deepest discouragement and when everything looked darkest for the cause she had at heart. As a result of her travels and speeches the foes of vice in every country united into a powerful federation.

THE ABOLITIONIST CONGRESS AT GENEVA. In 1877 this body, the International Federation for the Abolition of State Regulation of Vice, as it is now called, met at Geneva, five hundred strong and representing seventeen countries, and passed a notable series of resolutions under the sections into which the congress was organised.

SECTION ON HYGIENE. It was resolved (briefly stated) that self-control in the relation between the sexes is one of the indispensable bases of the health of the individual and the community:—that prostitution is a fundamental violation of the laws of health; that the true function of public hygiene is not only to supervise disease, but to do all that makes for public health, which is, in its highest expression, inseparable from public morality:—that all systems of "Morals Police" were complete failures and the medical examination revolting to human nature and worthless as a sanitary measure by reason of its inevitable incompleteness; that it was impossible for the most serious forms of venereal disease to be so discovered or prevented and that it gave a false guarantee of the health of the women subjected to it.

SECTION ON MORALITY. Resolved that license is as reprehensible in men as in women:—that the regulation of prostitution destroys the idea of the unity of the moral law:—that in regulating vice the state forgets its duty to afford protection equally to both sexes, degrades women and incites youth to evil:—that the system of licensed houses raises prostitution to the rank of a profession and sanctions the immoral doctrine that debauch is a necessity for men.

SECTION ON SOCIAL ECONOMY. Exposed the whole condition of the economic dependency of women, and traced it to the inequality established by law between men and women, pointing to the unequal wages and sex slavery of women as proofs of their charges.

SECTION ON LEGISLATION. Resolved that the regulation of prostitution lowered women to the grade of chattels, putting them beyond the pale of the law and inducing the state to violate its own penal code and forget its duty of giving protection to the young.

DECLINE OF MEDICAL SUPPORT OF REGULATION. The congress of 1874 seemed to mark the highest point of medical advocacy of regulation, and at the medical congresses of 1876 and 1877 the subject was not allowed to come up, as it became known that fearless and determined antagonists would appear. At a Regulationist congress in 1894, only three supporters of the "Morals Police" were present.

It would be interesting and useful to know just how much of the change in the medical attitude has been due to the influence of women physicians. From the time of the entrance of the heroic Elizabeth Blackwell and her sister Emily into this hitherto conservative profession, such women have consistently and steadily presented the nobler and more ethical—more spiritual—aspect of the questions relating to sex physiology and hygiene. Elizabeth Blackwell early declared, in a letter to her sister, her determination not to be intimidated or discouraged in the difficult task of attacking the social evil by methods of education, and her books and addresses on this subject are classics in their dignity and nobility of position. She was the first to address herself to parents. In 1852 she wrote to them of the Laws of Life in relation to girls, and in 1880 she wrote to them: "The fact must be clearly perceived and accepted that male chastity is a fundamental virtue in a State; that it secures the chastity of women, on which the moral qualities of fidelity, humanity, and trust depend, and that it secures the strength and truth of men, on which the intellectual vigour and wise government of a state depend."

From that time on women physicians as an entire body have stood unitedly for a single standard of morals and for the education of the public. In their ranks there can be found no division or opposing opinions on this subject. They are active in the warfare against vice, in every country where medicine has opened its doors to women, and, in our own country, they have been publicly called upon by their colleagues in the medical profession to carry the teachings of hygiene to the women of the land. Such women as Mary Putnam Jacobi, Sarah Hackett Stevenson, and Annie Daniels have brought medical science into perfect harmony with the most advanced civic standards, and their influence will be lasting.

THE FIRST AND SECOND CONFERENCES FOR THE PROPHYLAXIS OF SYPHILIS AND THE VENEREAL DISEASES. In 1899, the first international conference of important medical men and laymen met under this name in Brussels, and the second conference followed in the same city in 1902. An English writer says of the proceedings of these two weighty bodies that they marked the reconciliation of justice and morals with science.

The first conference took up six questions for discussion; they were: I. Systems of regulation now in force;—have they an influence on the frequency and the dissemination of syphilis and other venereal diseases? II. Medical supervision of prostitution;—is it capable of improvement? III. Tolerated houses;—is there, from the strictly medical point of view, any advantage in maintaining them, or is it better to suppress them? IV. Police supervision;—how to improve it. V. Number of women entering upon a life of prostitution;—how to decrease it. VI. What general propaganda could be made against prostitution?

Although much difference of opinion as to "regulation and control" was found to exist, as the discussions went on the following conclusions shaped themselves and were generally admitted.

1. The intervention of public powers in regulation as it exists has not given results of a certain or sufficient efficacy.

2. The prostitution of minor girls is most dangerous and should be the object of the most radical measures.

3. Better university instruction in venereology is needed.

4. The public power should be used to teach and to disseminate a knowledge of prostitution.

5. There should be a uniform system of statistics of prostitution and venereal diseases for all countries.

Disregarding all points on which there was

an absence of unanimity, the conference passed a set of eight resolutions which were, in brief, as follows:

RESOLUTIONS OF THE FIRST BRUSSELS CONFERENCE. 1. All governments shall be called upon to suppress absolutely prostitution among minors. 2. Societies of Sanitary and Moral Prophylaxis should be formed in every country. 3. It is the duty of governments to promote, by complete and compulsory university courses, the instruction of truly competent medical specialists in venereal diseases. 4. Moral teaching should be provided for orphans. 5. The utmost rigour of the law should be applied to men who live upon the profits of prostitution (cadets, *souteneurs*, etc.). 6. Each country should appoint a commission to study conditions, investigate the number of hospital beds, dispensaries, and other opportunities for free treatment that are available. 7. Education in sex morality should be offered to the public. 8. There should be a uniform method of statistics adopted in all countries alike, as a basis of correct data for the combat against venereal diseases.

THE SECOND BRUSSELS CONFERENCE. The

conference of 1902 discussed public prophylaxis under the following heads:

A.—As to prostitution—what legal measures are advisable? I. The general protection of minors of both sexes. II. The improvement of public medical relief, hospital dispensaries, etc. III. Contagion:—by midwives; in obstetrics generally; in shops and factories; by instruments; as arising in the management of employment agencies and intelligence offices; as related to the policing of hotels and lodgings.

B.—A penal code for the transmission of venereal disease; should one be adopted?

The subject of private prophylaxis was considered under the two following heads: I. How to teach the public and especially the young. II. How to improve the public medical service.

Statistics and special communications closed the sessions. This second conference and indeed both were very remarkable not only for the facts brought out, but also as showing, along with the rapidly advancing tendency of the best medical thought to think in unison with social moralists on this question, two things especially: one, the immense handicap of involuntary, unconscious sex dominance and egotism to men discussing these problems: the other, the conspicuous ignorance of many great medical specialists in matters of sociology. It is a mistake to suppose that an eminent authority in one line will be equally eminent as an authority in another. As a matter of fact, the general esteem and confidence proffered to the medical profession by the public has sometimes encouraged its members to believe that their pronouncements on social conditions are as final as their definitions of medical knowledge. This has been pointed out by various critics of the proceedings of the two conferences at Brussels.

Dr. Pileur, an advocate of regulation, admitted that the diversity of opinion on this point was so great as to amount to anarchy. He would allow adult women to practise prostitution with the agreement of three [men] commissioners, and would hold them to strict rules, punishing them for infraction thereof. In his plan no men are to be punished.

That was his theory: his facts are impressive. He urges the reduction of prostitution to an irreducible minimum, and believes that cutting off the minors will bring this about. He states that seventy-five per cent. of all prostitution begins before the age of twenty-one; further, that of these minor girls fifty per cent. are afflicted with venereal disease and twenty-five per cent. have syphilis. These figures, he holds, are understated and would be higher if investigation could be thorough and precise. He judges by the statistics of such girls as had been finally arrested in Paris as "clandestines," of whom seventy-two per cent. were found to be diseased when arrested. He holds that the prostitution of minors is the absolutely capital fact in the question of prostitution and insists that if all under twenty-one could be kept out, the number of women choosing the life, who might be called "chronic" or "persevering" prostitutes, would be surprisingly small. From a medical standpoint, he considers older women as less liable to disease, and estimates the amount of syphilis among them as seventeen per cent.

Dr. Neisser stated that the unanimous testimony of all nations was that irregular intercourse, especially that of prostitution, was the main source of all ravages by venereal diseases. The three factors in prostitution that are fatal in the hygienic sense are: Frequency of sex relations; absence of choice among persons; constant variety of persons. Prostitution is the knot around which contamination centres. Individual immoral relations are less dangerous, and, if infection then occurs, it has been accidentally introduced from prostitution. Nevertheless, he advocated the recognition and toleration of prostitution as a trade, unavoidable under present social conditions, and believes that it strengthens the control of the police over thieves and criminals to have the management of prostitution within their jurisdiction. After expounding this last-mentioned curious social view, he advocated teaching the principle of chastity to young men.

Henri Minod, an uncompromising abolitionist, quoted from many sources to show that real depravity is not a serious cause of prostitution. Few women find any enjoyment in this life. They regard it, not as pleasure, but as "work." M. Minod quoted some statistics of Dr. Le Pileur, to show the ages at which 582 girls were drawn into prostitution.

AGES AT WHICH GIRLS WERE RUINED:

6 were ruined when from 10–11 years old.
2 " " " " 11–12 " "
8 " " " " 12–13 " "
24 " " " " 13–14 " "

       50 were ruined when from 14–15 years old.
      142   "   "   "   " 15–16   "   "
      106   "   "   "   " 16–17   "   "
       86   "   "   "   " 17–18   "   "
       67   "   "   "   " 18–19   "   "
       38   "   "   "   " 19–20   "   "
       24   "   "   "   " 20–21   "   "
       11   "   "   "   " 21–22   "   "
       11   "   "   "   " 22–23   "   "
        3   "   "   "   " 23–24   "   "
        1 was   "   "   " 24–25   "   "
        3 were   "   "   " 25–26   "   "

[A set of figures corroborative of these, though not presented at the conference, are added here as being germane to the heading. They are given by the Rev. G. P. Merrick, in his *Work Among the Fallen*.

         11 ruined before 11 years of age.
         36   "   "   12   "   "   "
         62   "   "   13   "   "   "
        104   "   "   14   "   "   "
        358   "   "   15   "   "   "
      1,192   "   "   16   "   "   "
      1,425   "   "   17   "   "   "
      1,369   "   "   18   "   "   "
      1,158   "   "   20   "   "   "
        947   "   "   21   "   "   "
        703   "   "   22   "   "   "

He also makes statements that agree with those

of M. Minod, viz., that out of 100,000 cases personally known to him he had not found one hundred who did not loathe the life. Drink, said he, was a necessity to nerve them to endure it.]

Certain ones of the members of the conference of 1902 advocated laws making the transmission of venereal disease a penal offence. The weak points of this proposal were forcibly presented by Miss Blanche Leppington, of England, who pointed out: I. Danger of unjust accusation; II. Opportunities for blackmail; III. Dangers of publicity; IV. Avoidance of such retaliation by the self-respecting and its exploitation by the vile; V. Resultant estrangement of patients from physicians; VI. Resultant fostering of quackery.

Careful reading of the full proceedings leaves the settled conviction that the advocates of toleration and regulation have a weak case, contradict themselves and one another, and grasp wildly at the most absurd social remedies; while the abolitionists are logical, rational, unanimous, and show some knowledge of human nature and of social conditions. Again avoiding all controversial themes, the second conference agreed unanimously on the following resolutions: That there should be full, adequate, free hospital treatment for all cases of venereal disease; that patients should not be regarded as guilty persons, but simply as patients; that teaching in sex hygiene should be given to soldiers; that the education of the public should be continued and that emphasis should be laid on the doctrine that the health of young men is improved by continence; that uniform statistics should be kept; that the physiology of sex should be taught in the schools of all countries to the children of all ages. This done, the conference adjourned without fixing a date for reassembling, leaving the societies that had been formed at its instigation to carry on the work in their own countries.

THE SOCIETIES OF SANITARY AND MORAL PROPHYLAXIS. Among these national societies newly formed to carry on educational missions in regard to venereal diseases, the American Society of Sanitary and Moral Prophylaxis, under the presidency of its founder, Dr. Prince A. Morrow of New York City, stands easily in the lead by reason of its singleness of purpose (certain others still wrestling with the vexed question of regulation), the unassailable dignity of its tone in promulgating a teaching which harmonises the soundest medical science with a high morality, and its resultant widespread influence. Its membership is open to men and women, to the professions and to the laity, and this association, as well as the State Societies to which it has given the impulse, offers the needed opportunity for all who desire to ally themselves with the new crusade for the attainment of the single moral standard and the extirpation of the diseases of immorality.

REGULATION PASSING FROM THE CONTINENT. The reports of the Brussels Conference show that regulation is being discredited in the countries where it has long been under trial. Norway abolished the Morals Police in 1888, and since then the Norwegian women have defeated provisions that they believed portended a return to regulation.

Denmark and Sweden both reported a probable early cessation of police control with retention of medical inspection only. Italy has abolished regulation.

France has had two government commissions studying the subject; one, appointed in 1901, had no results. The second, appointed in 1903, upon which one woman was placed, gave a verdict of banishment for regulation; decided that prostitution is not a legal offence coming under the penal law, but is a social phenomenon to be combated, but not with force; agreed that it should be made punishable to "procure" even adults, even with their own consent, and framed a number of resolutions looking to a rational and humane discouragement of prostitution as a business, as well as to the treatment of venereal diseases. Their conclusions have not yet been enacted into legislation, but the force of public opinion will probably soon prevail over the small group of determined regulationists who still resist them.

DANGER OF REGULATION NOT PAST. In spite of all the available testimony against it, tolerated and licensed vice still finds advocates. Arguments in its favour have been advanced, and efforts made to introduce regulation systems in this country. Doubtless such efforts will be repeated, from time to time, and it is therefore most important that the moral public should be well grounded in the lessons taught by English and continental experience, and ready to make intelligent resistance to any such attempted invasion.[1]

[1] See Appendix A.

There have always been, and perhaps always will be, some honest and well-intentioned apologists for regulation. The existing writings and speeches made by members of this class, however, such as may be found in the transactions of a society organised in England during the crusade against the Contagious Diseases Acts, whose aim was to support regulation, show, alongside of perfectly good intentions, an extreme mediocrity of intelligence, a very limited point of view, and a profound ignorance of their subject. Such banal opinions as that erring girls would find, in the police, wise and benevolent friends, who would lead them back to their families; and that inscribed women would become so accustomed to the routine of their supervised lives as to miss it if discontinued, show sufficiently the worth of their information.

On the other hand, all accounts teem with evidence of the disastrous results of regulatory legislation, and this evidence will now be summed up, at the risk of a certain amount of repetition, in order to bring all the arguments of the opposition into one place.

BRUTALISING EFFECT OF REGULATION ON

CHARACTER. A terrible revelation is that of the brutalising effect of regulatory enactments upon the natures of those who administer and enforce them. This was strikingly shown in all the evidence laid before the Select Committee in England, and appears again in the reports of the Brussels conferences. Officers of the army and military surgeons were seen to have reverted to the brute; as in the case of the one who ordered an establishment for his regiment in advance, and, knowing well that many would be little girls, excused this on the ground that "In India prostitution begins in the cradle": and of the other, who granted permits for licensed houses. A menacing disregard for the good of the civil community was suggested in the testimony of such men, that "diseased women, if incurable, were expelled from the cantonment." But, it was asked,—where did they go? For, unless they could die at once, they must go somewhere and be a danger to their environment.

Equally disturbing evidence of the decline of traditional chivalry under the effects of the supervision of vice is at-hand in the suggestion of a German surgeon, who, angered by the failure of inscribed women to appear regularly for examination, would have had them whipped for absence; and in that of a French doctor who proposed imprisoning each woman for several days before examination, in order to prevent their tampering with symptoms. The quarrels and disputes between medical and police supervisors have also been numerous and undignified.

In reading such material, one feels keenly that the supervision of vice degrades the medical profession to a plane little higher than that of the cadet or *souteneur*.

THE INSULT TO RELIGION. The insult to religion was deadly. There was (and still is) a wide-spread belief in distant provinces that licensed prostitution was a part of the Christian religion. The editor of *The Sentinel* pointed out the incongruity of ordinances passed "in the year of our LORD" for licensing vice, and Mrs. Butler, in her evidence, said, "Few things shock the sense of the country more than the fact that religious teaching is allied with state regulation of vice." Even as late as 1908 the statement appeared in an English journal that one reason for an outbreak of syphilis in an African province was "the introduction of Christianity."

THE SANITARY INEFFICIENCY OF REGULATION. The entire mass of testimony makes it clear that state regulation, licensing, and medical examination does not diminish venereal disease. Conflicting and contradictory columns of statistics do not alter this conclusion. Dr. Mounier of Utrecht says that statistical methods are futile in the clearing up of disputes as to the efficacy of regulation. Figures showing results favourable to regulation were based on imperfect knowledge. One prominent error, made before the discovery of the *Spirochæte pallida*, was in the confusing of venereal ulcer with syphilis. The difference between them was not understood. Remembering that venereal ulcer is the least serious and most readily cured of the venereal diseases, it will at once be clear that its figures might easily show an improvement which, if credited to the graver disease, would be most misleading. Again, remembering the variable period of inoculation of the *Spirochæte pallida*, and the latency of the *gonococcus*, possibilities of error are evidently many. Still another source of error lay here: it has been found that syphilis shows a certain variability when observed over long periods of time, having its epochs of increase and decrease.

This obscure and, to many, unknown phenomenon makes observations over short time-periods of little value.

The reasons for the sanitary failure of regulation may be tabulated as follows:

I. THE ONE-SIDED EXAMINATION. It is surprising that the plan of examining women only while men were unexamined should ever have been advanced as worthy of being taken seriously. Morrow says of this: "The prostitute is but the purveyor of the infection;—she simply returns to her male partner, the prostituant, as he is called, the infection which she has received from another prostituant. In the ultimate analysis it will be found that the male is the chief malefactor." Again he says: "The health officer of a port might as well attempt to prevent the importation of infectious disease from a plague-infested vessel by quarantining the infected women while permitting the infected men to go free." This weakness has been admitted in official circles, and Neisser and others at the conference of 1902 advocated examining every man who entered a house of ill-fame. The naïveté of this suggestion speaks for itself. Men would not submit to it. This precaution has been tried occasionally in armies and navies and has been rejected as a "degradation" involving "loss of respect" to the men.

II. LENGTH OF TIME BETWEEN EXAMINATIONS. The usual time of one or two weeks between examinations is too long. A woman may appear free from disease at one time and develop an infectious discharge before the next. This has also been recognised and more frequent examination recommended—even one or two weekly. But aside from the great expense to the taxpayers (many of whom are women) in supporting a staff large enough to make this everywhere possible, it is acknowledged that even the most enslaved women would rebel.

III. MEDIATE CONTAGION. Mechanical transmission of disease or "mediate contagion" is believed to be possible. The woman in this case, remaining uninfected herself, passes on to one man an infection which she has received from another.

IV. CLANDESTINE PROSTITUTION. The difficulty of the "clandestine" is perhaps the most obstinate of all. So great is the detestation of police and medical control among women that the greatest zeal and energy on the part of the officials cannot prevent numbers of them from practising secretly. While all medical authorities agree that these are the most dangerous prostitutes, the most unfaltering believers in regulation can give no suggestion for strengthening this weak link in the chain. This weakness has been realised in every country where regulation has been tried. Pontoppidan wrote in 1903 that 5000 women were inscribed by the police of Paris, in that year, while there were 50,000 clandestines. Figures for Berlin in 1896 were even worse; viz., 4039 women inscribed, while the number of clandestines equalled that of Paris. Dr. Käthe Schirmacher has recently stated that the police of Paris, in the last thirty years, had arrested 725,000 women and had inscribed 155,000. Twenty-five per cent. of those inscribed, she added, had disappeared.

V. REGULATION INCREASES VICE. Ample testimony is at hand to show that immoral practices increase with the sense of security imparted by official inspection. In the words of Dr. C. Bell Taylor, there is "multiplied indulgence springing from the apparent immunity." In armies it has been understood that the government purposed providing the regiments with "clean girls," and in civil communities young men speak openly of the advantages of licensed houses. The more wide-spread immoral practices are, the greater of course must be the danger of infection.

VI. IGNOMINY ATTACHES TO TREATMENT. Under regulation the ignominy attaching to the compulsory treatment deters respectable patients from seeking medical aid; brings the special hospital into disrepute and fosters the industry of quacks, who offer secrecy and regard for the sensitive pride of the individual. The seriousness of this danger is widely recognised.

Pontoppidan, after a moderate and rational review of the whole subject, says: "Control is entirely without positive value as a security."

IMMORAL NATURE OF REGULATION. Aside from sanitary inefficiency, regulation stands condemned on the following counts:

1. It corrupts and demoralises the police and offers endless opportunities for blackmail and extortion. Here it may be emphasised that, although there is in the United States no

legal regulation of vice, yet there is blackmail and extortion because the police, under the pressure of corrupt social elements have developed a system of protection for vice which approaches closely to an official alliance with it.

2. It exposes innocent women to persecution. Numerous instances of this kind are on record. Respectable girls have been reported to the police from motives of revenge or jealousy, and self-supporting women have been driven from positions and their property manipulated away from them. Cases have been known where such victims have been driven to suicide.

3. That it perpetuates a class of women who are deprived of the protection of the law has been referred to. For such women, no matter what their just grievance, justice in the courts would be a thing unheard of. Even without regulation it is doubtful whether legal justice exists for these unfortunates.

4. Regulation bears with special hardship on the poorest women. Indeed, it may be said that only the very poor and defenceless are exposed to its full horrors. The fact that immoral women who are able to command ample means are safe against the severities of the law has been

frequently mentioned by writers belonging to different countries.

5. It puts governments in the position of endorsing the assumption that women may be sacrificed for men's pleasure. It even tends to make it appear that women are the chief offenders and the primary corrupting influence, and may therefore be treated with a disregard of justice and decency. On this point M. Jules Favre said: "The worst that could befall the public health is nothing to the corruption of morals and national life engendered, propagated, and prolonged by the system of official surveillance." Again, with regulation, the state is placed in a position not clearly different from that of the individual agents of immorality, and all taxpayers, women as well as men, are compelled to pay for the maintenance of officials to supervise prostitution. A German member of the Reichstag, speaking on this point, said: "The state which officially tolerates and guarantees houses of prostitution assumes the rôle of Procurer, a delinquent whom the German penal code punishes with imprisonment and hard labour."

6. It destroys respect for women and thus tends to make men unmanly and cowardly. And

the flourishing and unrestricted commercial prostitution which has been permitted to develop in the United States breeds this same contempt and unmanliness.

7. It blights that high ideal of parenthood and especially of motherhood that consecrates the functions of physical life. And the very existence of prostitution, regulated or unregulated, brings on this blight. No one has dwelt upon this truth more earnestly than Mrs. Butler. In her testimony before the Commons Committee she said:

> There is nothing in the physical being of a man that corresponds to the sacredness of the maternal functions in a woman, and these functions, and every organ connected with them, ought to be held in reverence by man. When this reverence ceases to be felt through the habitual outrage of any class of women, however degraded that class may already be, the demoralisation of society at large is sure to follow.

8. Finally, it is clear that the various systems of police protection and state licensing of prostitution have been the breeder and the main security of the most shocking of modern evils, the white slave traffic.

Systems of "segregation" deserve the same condemnation as regulation and for the same reasons.

CHAPTER II

THE WHITE SLAVE TRAFFIC

THAT this trade in girls for immoral purposes has grown naturally and inevitably out of the continental system of regulated vice is too evident to be contested. The existence of this traffic was at first undreamed of by Mrs. Butler and her associates, but they soon came into collision with it. In 1879, Mr. Alfred Dyer received information that a young English girl was detained against her will in a licensed house in Brussels, and intended committing suicide as the only escape. By the aid of a Belgian clergyman she was rescued, and then began a life and death struggle for the exposure of the evil. In time the British Society succeeded in obtaining the names of many men and women who were systematically engaged in this trade in London, as well as the addresses of fifty licensed houses in France, Belgium, and Holland, to which the girls were sold. They also succeeded in exposing all the methods and practices in the trade. It was shown that the exculpatory statements of the police were false in every particular; that girls were decoyed under pretence of obtaining employment, and that there were systematic methods of intimidation. It was proved that girls were asked in foreign tongues whether they came willingly, and then, not understanding, or thinking they were entering domestic service, they were inscribed as having come of their own free will. Again, they were listed under false names and then threatened with imprisonment for "forgery" if they rebelled. All street clothes were taken from them. A skilful system involved them deeply in debt to their captors. If resistant, they were beaten and starved. Padded cells were found in the houses which were visited daily by the police, even the windows and doors being covered. It was also shown that the names, persons, and pursuits of the foreign agents in England were perfectly well known to the police and had been so for years, but "the state of the English law did not authorise" their arrest or extradition. As investigations went deeper the traffic in England was traced back to the year 1857.

The experience gained in this crusade led Mrs. Butler to say:

As an inevitable and necessary accompaniment of the establishment of licensed houses of prostitution under government patronage all over the world, there exists the most extensive slave traffic in the interests of vice. This fact has become . . . fully acknowledged during the last few years.

In a memorandum to the Committee of the House of Lords M. de Laveleye wrote:

The white slave traffic is carried on . . . and will not be suppressed as long as prostitution constitutes, on the continent, a traffic, not only tolerated but legalised, privileged, and licensed in the same way as any other traffic. The legal organisation of debauchery is the chief support of the odious trade against which we are seeking a remedy. . . . This state of things, which places prostitution on the footing of a recognised commerce, must naturally produce a most dire effect on the police and on all who are brought into contact with these abominable institutions. . . . The traffic in women, that is to say, the letting on hire of human beings for debauchery, as of horses and other cattle, is a system contrary to all morality and all sense of right and ought to be universally forbidden. As long as these establishments remain legalised institutions, the traffic which supplies them will not be stopped.

THE SHARE OF LAW IN THE WHITE SLAVE

TRAFFIC. The members of the British Society were not long in discovering how much the laws of the country had to do with the extent and the security of the trade in girls. Briefly stated, the features of the laws relating to the protection of girls were, at that time, as follows: To abduct a girl under twenty-one for immoral purposes was a felony, if she belonged to a propertied class or family. If she was propertyless, it was only a misdemeanour to abduct her under sixteen. Thus a penniless girl, sixteen years old, could be lawfully decoyed for immoral purposes, as she could claim no protection from the state or its agents the police. (And here again let it be recalled that women wage-earners and women taxpayers were helping to provide the public funds needed for maintaining such legislation.) But still worse was the discovery that girls having neither parents nor guardians might safely be abducted even under sixteen, as the law provided no penalty at all for such act, nor any protection for such girls. Here was obviously a deliberate and intentional legal omission devised by legislators with the sole and single purpose of maintaining a supply of victims,—not, perhaps, for the white slave trade, but for the institution of prostitution.

This cannot be too plainly stated. Such careful legal fencing could not be accidental; and that it was indeed not accidental was fully proved, later, by the long and stubborn resistance of the lawmakers to any amendment.

Another strange feature of these strangely unchivalrous laws, was that a father, having reason to believe, but not possessing legal proof, that his daughter was in a house of prostitution, could not secure a search-warrant to look for her, nor could any benevolent friend do so.

FACTS LEARNED OF THE TRADE IN GIRLS. The following facts were brought out as to the trade in girls: girls between sixteen and twenty were the most desirable, because the most docile.

It was important to entrap only healthy girls, as, if any were found to be diseased and to require hospital care, the trade lost money.

A skilled system of falsehood was practised in order to evade the fairly strict laws of continental countries relating to minors.

The police were always in sympathy and sometimes in guilty complicity with the agents and the tolerated houses. One European police official explained their attitude thus: "We cannot injure establishments legally authorised and in which so much capital is vested." The English committee declared: "Reliance on the police has misled all who have trusted to it."

Intelligence offices, all licensed, were the main avenues of the trade. The girls were called "colis" (packages) and the business was perfectly organised, with routes, ports, agents, and travellers; cargoes and technical phraseology, prices and values all worked out.

English birth certificates (false) were bought for a small sum.

Four fifths of the girls so enslaved were orphans.

A close relation was found to exist between the city authorities and keepers or owners of tolerated houses. The first exposure in Brussels implicated the mayor and two aldermen, all of whom resigned.

THE STRUGGLE FOR IMPROVED LEGISLATION. The history of the attempts made to amend these laws is highly instructive, as showing the different points of view of the governed and the governing, and the opposition of interests between enfranchised men and unenfranchised women.

The Society sent a memorial to the proper minister in 1880 asking for a deputation to be received. A year went by without answer. On making a second appeal, the committee were informed that official inquiry had been made and it had been found that the Society had overstated the case. A petition signed by 1000 women was then presented by Mrs. Butler in 1881. An inquiry by the House of Lords followed. Two years later the Lords reported, making various recommendations for the better protection of girls. The House of Lords passed these measures, and the House of Commons defeated them. The same thing was repeated in 1884. In 1885 a third bill, in which the "age of consent" was set at fifteen years, was about to be killed in the House of Commons, when the *Pall Mall Gazette*[1] brought out its revelations which aroused the public wrath and drove the legislators to act.

THE WHITE SLAVE TRAFFIC IN THE UNITED STATES. As the revelations of the international traffic in young girls were unfolded, leaders of communities formed National Vigilance Leagues to carry on a war of extermination against it. There are now Leagues in Great Britain, Germany, France, Russia, Sweden, Norway, Belgium, Hol-

[1] July 10, 1885.

land, Italy, Spain, Portugal, Switzerland, Austria, and the United States, the latter having been formed in 1906 with O. Edward Janney, M.D., of Baltimore, as its president. These Leagues have brought about an international agreement by which the governments of the countries represented bind themselves to a concerted action in suppression of the white slave trade. In 1907, Congress passed an act designed to crush the traffic in foreign girls, as the limitations of the constitution of the United States confine its jurisdiction to immigrants. This act provided that any person who should keep, maintain, support, or harbour any alien woman for immoral purposes within three years after her arrival in this country should be punishable for misdemeanour by five years' imprisonment or $5000 fine. The federal government has no power over traffic in American women, carried on within the States themselves.

In the process of enforcing the law regarding aliens the United States District Attorney at Chicago was directed to take the proper steps for securing the conviction of certain persons who were suspected of violating the statute. The raids upon houses of prostitution and arrests of their inmates that were made with this end in view brought to light a mass of evidence of a terrible, much of an unspeakable nature, and the District Attorney, Edwin W. Sims, and his assistant, H. D. Parkin, as well as convicting a number of procurers, felt it their duty to make known to American parents the conditions imperilling their daughters, as it was evident that a profound state of ignorance prevailed as to the existence in our country of so vile a trade. They therefore wrote a series of articles for a popular magazine in which the facts they had learned were most clearly and explicitly stated. Their investigations led them to believe that some 65,000 American girls and 15,000 aliens are being entrapped yearly for the white slave trade. The methods by which they are taken vary: promises of employment, bogus messages, plausible invitations, deceptive marriage ceremonies, even real marriage. The runaway marriage is a device frequently used with country girls of American families. The District Attorney believed that there was a syndicate which carried on a business in the ruin of girls as steady, regular, and systematic as any great business of a legitimate kind, and that its ramifications extended to the Pacific with distributing centres in nearly all the large cities. Recent Congressional commissions of inquiry believe that no definite syndicate exists, but that there is a general understanding between the agents in different cities. This is, of course, equally menacing and serious, and does not relieve the situation of its darkness.

Of the details of the life, Sims repeats almost the very words of the English investigators into the Brussels conditions. He writes:

When a white slave is sold and landed in a house or dive she becomes a prisoner . . . in each of these places is a room having but one door, to which the keeper holds the key. Here are locked all the street clothes, shoes, and ordinary apparel . . . the finery provided for the girls is of a nature to make their appearance on the street impossible. Then, in addition to this handicap, the girl is placed at once in debt to the keeper for a wardrobe . . . she cannot escape while she is in debt, and she can never get out of debt. . . . Not many of the women in this class expect to live more than ten years—perhaps the average is less. Many die painful deaths by disease [venereal] many by consumption, but it is hardly beyond the truth to say that suicide is their general expectation. . . . The facts that I have stated are for the awakening of parents and guardians of girls.

Among the individual instances described by

the District Attorney was that of a little girl who was fourteen years old when stolen, and who, besides being used as a scrubwoman by day, in two and one half years' time had been compelled to earn eight thousand dollars for her owner.

The statement made at the Brussels conference, that the number of chronic or persevering prostitutes, if separated from the others, would be surprisingly small, is borne out by Sims's declaration that only about twenty per cent. of all prostitutes are willingly such, or have chosen or preferred the life, while all the other eighty per cent. have either been forced into it by poverty and destitution, or have been betrayed, trapped, enticed, or sold into it.

The National Vigilance League has published a pamphlet called *The Nation and the Traffic in Women*, addressed to the American people, in which ample facts as to the present situation are set forth with moderation and as entire absence of sensationalism as the extraordinary truth permits.

The facts speak for themselves, and the ultimate responsibility for these conditions, in an unscrupulous use of property, and in the protection secured for vice by corrupt sordid elements of society who have been permitted to seize the machinery of government for their own evil and mercenary purposes, is laid squarely where it belongs, at the doors of the business community and respectable citizens of the country.

Mention is made of a city "where the authorities seem to regard the slavery of young girls as a part of the legitimate business of the city." Of another, where the money to build slave pens was furnished by the business men of the town. Procurers of young girls, it is pointed out, "are useful to the politicians, and, when arrested, escape through political influence—while smart lawyers are employed to defend them when arrested."

The hopes of dealing an effectual blow to the white slave trade were painfully frustrated by the decision of the Supreme Court of the United States early in 1909, which set free the traders, accused by the federal authorities, on the ground of the unconstitutionality of that clause in the immigration law under which they were prosecuted. This leaves the future status of white slave traders to the slow and uncertain action of the legislatures of the States of the Union, many of which, it has been found, have failed entirely to provide adequate protection for young girls.[1]

THE LAWS OF PROTECTION FOR GIRLS IN THE UNITED STATES. How high the standards of the States are likely to be may be conjectured from the provisions of those laws designed to give protection to girls, which are commonly known as the laws of the age of consent.

This age, beyond which there is no legal protection for girls against seduction and violation of the person, nor punishment for men committing such acts, was originally fixed by the common law at TEN YEARS.

No American State took any steps toward raising this age until 1864. From that time to the present, the insistent urging of women has brought about some gradual amendment, though, with the fixing of a higher age limit, the corresponding penalties have usually been reduced, and thirteen States name no penalty at all for violation of the law. The following data are taken from the *History of Woman Suffrage*, by Susan B. Anthony and Ida Husted Harper, and are there carried up

---

[1] The federal law of 1910 which, at the time of writing, is before Congress, has not had time to prove its effectiveness.

to the year 1900. It has been thought best to retain that year as a dividing line, and leave changes made since that time for mention in future revisions.

Three States then had the age of ten years fixed as the age of protection against rape. They were Florida, Georgia, and Mississippi. Florida, however, recognised two grades of protection: the age of consent (ten), and the age of protection (sixteen at first, later raised to eighteen). Certain details will be given on a subsequent page.

Two States, Kentucky and West Virginia, gave protection up to twelve years. One, New Hampshire, to thirteen years. Ten, Alabama, Illinois, Indiana, Maine, Missouri, Nevada, New Mexico, South Carolina, Virginia, Wisconsin, to fourteen years. Two, Iowa and Texas, to fifteen years. Nineteen, Arkansas, California, Connecticut, Dakota, District of Columbia, Louisiana, Maryland, Massachusetts, Michigan, Minnesota, Montana, New Jersey, Ohio, Oregon, Pennsylvania, Rhode Island, Tennessee, Vermont, Washington to sixteen years. Nine, Arizona, Colorado, Delaware, Idaho, Kansas, Nebraska, New York, Utah, Wyoming, to eighteen years.

Some brief account of the ways in which

amendments to these laws have been brought about will be instructive as showing that it is not easy to improve them.

Arkansas raised the protected age from twelve to sixteen in 1893. But the penalty, which had previously been not less than five years nor more than twenty-five, was reduced to one year.

In California the Women's Christian Temperance Union asked the legislature in 1887 to raise the protected age from ten (as it then was) to eighteen. The legislature raised it to fourteen. In 1895 the women secured an amendment fixing it at eighteen. The governor vetoed it. In 1897 the women tried again, and secured a bill fixing sixteen as the protected age; this was finally passed and became law.

Dakota raised the age from ten to fourteen in 1887. In 1895, the women of Dakota tried to obtain legislation fixing the age at eighteen, but only succeeded in getting sixteen years enacted into law. Moreover the penalty was lowered and the following clause introduced:

No conviction can be had in case the female is over ten years and the man under the age of twenty and if it appears to the satisfaction of the jury that the female was sufficiently matured and informed to understand the nature of the act and to consent thereto.

In Delaware the age of *seven years only* was legally protected against the brutality of man until 1889. In that year the women of the State petitioned the legislature and secured fifteen years, but the penalties were lowered and no minimum penalty was fixed. In 1895 the women brought another plea and obtained eighteen years. It is, however, very difficult to secure convictions and in cases where men have been convicted they have been pardoned.

In Florida, the women of the Christian Temperance Union made many attempts to have the age of consent and of protection both raised, from, respectively, ten and sixteen years to eighteen. Their bills were always laid on the table. In 1901, they made a valiant effort with two bills: the one, raising the age of protection against rape from ten to fourteen, passed the House but was lost in the Senate; the other, raising the age of protection from sixteen to eighteen, was finally forced through by a small majority and in the face of all manner of obstructive devices, but no minimum penalty was attached to it. The age of protection against rape remained at ten years, with loopholes for the evasion of the penalty.

In Georgia, the suffrage association of Atlanta tried to raise the protected age from ten to eighteen. The bill was killed in committee. In 1899, the attempt was again made. The Women's Christian Temperance Union also came forward, asking for twenty-one years. A bill raising the age to twelve was brought in and defeated. Reconsidered at the plea of the women, it was re-defeated more emphatically.

In Indiana, bills urged by women to raise the age above fourteen have never been permitted to come out of committee.

Iowa amended her law in 1886, raising the age from ten to thirteen. In 1896, the Women's Christian Temperance Union secured an advance to fifteen, with heavy penalty, but a clause provides that the man cannot be convicted on the testimony of the injured person without corroborative testimony.

In Kansas, immediately after women obtained municipal suffrage, the age of consent was raised from ten to eighteen years. The law of Colorado was also carried by the women's vote in their first year of exercising the franchise.

Michigan raised the age of consent from ten to fourteen in 1887. In 1895, an amendment to eighteen was introduced and passed, but the day after the friends of the bill, thinking it safe, had gone home, it was reconsidered and changed to sixteen.

Minnesota altered the age from ten to sixteen in 1891. Thousands of women had petitioned in vain for eighteen.

New York raised its protected age for girls in 1887 from ten years to sixteen. A few years later there was an attempt made to reduce it to twelve. The women made themselves heard in indignant protest and the effort was relinquished. In 1895 the age of eighteen was legally secured. It is, however, almost impossible to secure convictions and many flagrant cases of assault on little girls go unpunished, the writer's long experience as a district nurse having brought a number of such cases to her personal knowledge, where the miscreants have been sheltered behind political and police protection.

It is natural to wonder what arguments men can find for defending such standards on the floors of legislatures: this has been answered by Dr. Elizabeth Blackwell from English history, and

American records show the same reasons given. One is, the need of protecting men against blackmail for false charges, and the other, the physical fact of the early oncoming of puberty in little girls. That it is possible for a child of twelve to become pregnant has seemed to legislators of this type reason enough for regarding her as a matured woman.

SOURCES OF MATERIAL USED IN THE PREPARATION OF PART II

American Society of Moral and Sanitary Prophylaxis. Transactions. All volumes.

Amos, Sheldon, A Comparative Survey of Laws in Force for the Prohibition, Regulation, and Licensing of Vice in England and other Countries. London, 1877.

Blaschko, A., Syphilis und Prostitution vom Standpunkte der öffentlichen Gesundheitspflege. Berlin, 1893.

Booth, C., The Iniquity of State-Regulated Vice. London, 1884.

British Committee of the I. F. A. S. R. V. The Shield. London.

Brussels. Conférence Internationale pour le Prophylaxie de la Syphilis et des Maladies Venériennes. 1899.

———, The same. Second Conference, 1902.

Butler, Josephine E., A Grave Question. London, 1885 or 1886.

Butler, Josephine E., Personal Reminiscences of a Great Crusade. London, 1896.

Butler, Josephine E., Principles of the Abolitionists. London, 1885.

Butler, Josephine E., The Revival and Extension of the Abolitionist Cause. London, 1887.

Committee of Fifteen, The, The Social Evil, with Special Reference to New York. New York, 1902.

Congrès des Sciences Médicales, Compte Rendu Résumé, Troisième Session, Vienne, 1873. Paris, 1876.

Dolléans, E., La Police des Mœurs. Paris, 1903.

Dyer, A. S., The European Slave Trade. London, 1880.

Dyer, A. S., The Slave Trade in European Girls to India. London, 1893.
Fiaux, F. L., La Police des Mœurs. Paris, 1888.
Geneva. Conférence du Genève, 1899. Fédération Abolitioniste Internationale. Compte Rendu. Geneva, 1900.
Guyot, Yves. Prostitution under the Regulation System, 1884.
House of Commons, Select Committee to Inquire into the Contagious Diseases Acts. Report, 3 vols., 1880, 1881, 1882.
House of Commons, Select Committee on the Contagious Diseases Acts. Minority Report. Reprinted from Parliamentary Papers, 340, Session of 1882.
House of Lords Committee, Prostitution in Hong Kong. (Parliamentary Paper C. 309.)
House of Lords Committee on the Law Relating to the Protection of Young Girls. Report, 1881. Appendix.
House of Lords Committee on the Law Relating to the Protection of Young Girls. Reports and Papers. Vol. ix.
Joest, Wilhelm, Du Japon en Allemagne par le Sibéria. [Routes, ports, cargoes, etc., of white slave trade.]
Ladies' National Association for the Abolition of Government Regulation of Vice. Publications, London.
Ladies' National Association for the Repeal of the Contagious Diseases Acts, Reports, Liverpool, 1871. Tracts on the Contagious Diseases Acts, 1871, 1883.
London Committee for Suppressing the Traffic in British Girls. Reports 1881, 1885, 1886.
McClure, S. S., The Tammanyising of a Civilisation. In McClure's Magazine, November, 1909.
Martineau, Harriet, Autobiography. Edited by M. W. Chapman, London, 1877.
Martineau, Harriet, Letters on State Regulation of Vice. In Daily News, 1859.
Scheven, Katharina, Denkschrift über die in Deutschland bestehenden Verhältnisse in Bezug auf das Bordellwesen. In Schriften des Bundes Deutscher Frauenvereine, Heft. VI., 1904.
Schirmacher, Käthe, M.D., The Work of the Extra-Parlia-

mentary Commission in France. Translated from Der Abolitionist. In "The Shield," October, 1909.

"Sentinel" Tracts. The Licensing of Sin in India.

Service de Sûreté publique et de Salubrité. Rapport. Brussels, 1880.

Stansfeld, Right Hon. James, M.P., The Failure of the Contagious Diseases Acts as Proved, etc., London.

Stansfeld, Right Hon. James, M.P., Lord Kimberley's Defence of the Government Brothel System, etc. 1882.

Stead, W. T., Josephine E. Butler: A Life Sketch. London, 1888.

Taylor, C. Bell, M.D., The Statistical Result of the Contagious Diseases Acts as Deduced from the Parliamentary Papers. 1872.

Turner, George Kibbe. The Daughters of the Poor. In McClure's Magazine, November, 1909.

White Slave Traffic. In Pall Mall Gazette, July, 1885.

Part III. The Prevention of Venereal Disease

CHAPTER I

UNDERLYING PRINCIPLES OF PREVENTION

PROSTITUTION TO BE PREVENTED. The genuine prevention of venereal disease is only made possible by the prevention of prostitution. Prostitution cannot be retained and the diseases fostered in it be eliminated. Prostitution must be rooted out, unless modern civilised states are content to look forward to the same fate which befell ancient Rome.

The English women, as they worked on through their crusade, came to see what at first they had not realised, that what they were making war upon was actually the social institution of prostitution itself. Thirty-five years ago Mrs. Butler said, in a public address: "That we are, and have been all along, contending for more than the mere repeal of these unjust and unholy Acts of Parliament, is proved by certain signs which are becoming more and more clear and frequent."

She went on: "We were perhaps ourselves unconscious—some of us are probably yet unconscious—how great is the undertaking upon which we have entered," and she then added with great solemnity, "it only very gradually dawned with perfect clearness on my mind that it is the old, the inveterate, the deeply-rooted evil of prostitution itself against which we are destined to make war." Mrs. Butler was saddened by seeing that some men, who had aided her against the special tyranny of special laws, grew cold and fell away as they found that her purpose struck at the very existence of prostitution itself. But her ideals of lofty personal and civic morality are now justified and sustained by those discoveries and teachings of science which, in her day, were still unheard, as to the causation and propagation of venereal diseases and even more so as to heredity. What men will not refrain from under persuasion alone, they will learn to refrain from under the warnings of medical and sanitary science, when these teachings are widely disseminated throughout all social circles. Just as the great mass of people have responded with readiness and intelligence to the doctrine of the preventability of tuberculosis, so, when they understand, will they respond to the doctrine of the far easier preventability of venereal diseases.

Even if the immoral projects of some writers could be realised in the use of immunising vaccines or serums to enable men to continue indulgence with greater security, venereal diseases would still continue to exist while prostitution exists, and, unless every man and woman in the world could be so vaccinated, there would be no security that the reckless, the unthinking, and the unsuspecting innocent would not continue to fall victims to, and to become carriers of, these deadly scourges. Nor is it credible that the aroused moral sense of humanity would consent to the general compulsory vaccination of syphilis and gonorrhœa as it does to that of smallpox, because moral sense, or even plain every-day common-sense, will distinguish between diseases which cannot be extirpated by moral living and the exertion of self-control through the power of the intelligent will, and diseases which can be so extirpated. The deliberate use of immunising substances with the intention of making it hygienically safe for men to continue a brutal misuse of women such as falls far below the practices of animals in vileness, could only be tolerated in a society that was ready for its own ruin. If such a practice is to be recommended as desirable for military recruits, and regarded as hopeful by military authorities, then this is only one more reason for the imperative social necessity of replacing the outworn military ideals by those of a higher conception of human brotherhood.[1]

However great may be the boon science has to bring to the present victims of immorality in the form of merciful antitoxins which may shear disease of its worst terrors, as diphtheria has been shorn by the serum of Behring, it will nevertheless remain true that real prevention does not rest there. Dr. Prince A. Morrow, president of the American Society of Sanitary and Moral Prophylaxis, says: "It is not a question of making prostitution safe, but of preventing the making of prostitutes." This lofty teaching is now being reiterated by ever larger numbers of the foremost leaders of medical science.

There are, in truth, no other diseases whose absolute prevention lies so wholly in human power as these.

[1] Various articles and books have been written on this line, which the author hesitates to mention because of the possibility of seeming to recommend them.

KNOWLEDGE IS ESSENTIAL. The first essential in a campaign of prevention is full, open, and serious instruction for all classes of society upon the situation as it exists to-day; instruction without exaggeration, but also without concealment, of the present extent of disease of venereal origin, and with the most emphatic and positive information upon the real source of danger in prostitution. It will be found that not only is the extent to which venereal diseases have been allowed to prey upon the national stock utterly undreamed of by great numbers of highly intelligent persons, but that their very existence is, to thousands of others, only the vaguest hearsay, while to thousands more absolutely unknown. Now, as in combating typhoid fever and the plague the first thing needful is that all shall know that there are such diseases, whence their origin, and how they may be cut off at their source, so it is essential that every citizen shall know that there are venereal diseases, where they arise, and how they may be exterminated.

Therefore, a wide-spread campaign of popular education must be the first movement made. This has already been begun by the national societies founded for the purpose, and, as their task is a most difficult one, they should have the active support of every right thinking man and woman. Extreme difficulties meet this movement at the outset, arising from the peculiarly personal origin of these diseases, the prevailing false modesty as to the reproductive functions, and the generally dense ignorance of the physiology and hygiene of the generative organs. The vulgar prudery and hypocrisy of a past age compelled all such subjects to be tabooed, as being indelicate or improper. Perhaps this point of view has been encouraged by those whose interests were selfish or evil; certainly nothing could better serve such interests than the veil of silence and the cloak of embarrassment drawn over subjects so vital, pertaining to functions by nature so sacred, but by man so horribly debased. The function of reproduction, for which the organs of generation have been evolved, though it has been dragged through the mire of vulgar thoughts and cruel abuse, is yet the noblest, as it should be the most held in reverence of all human powers. Reproduction is natural, and should no more be regarded vulgarly than are the changes of the seasons. It is a type and symbol of immortality. It is indeed a present and visible immortality, and its humble physical phenomena should never obscure its exalted significance. The generative act should only be performed in the sincerity of aspiration to bring a new being into the world. Such being the truth, the depravity of exercising so miraculous a power for the sole desire of a passing pleasure of sensation, often combining with it drunkenness, and orgies in which all human dignity and decency are cast away, is so complete that the decay and fall of nations would seem to need no further explanation.

The generative organs do not suffer by non-use. This statement is now being emphasised with great earnestness by our foremost medical teachers. Nor does the general health suffer by their non-use. This is also emphasised, and is the basis of the modern scientific teaching upon sex hygiene that is now being given to young men in the universities of many countries.

It must be seen to that no children are allowed to grow up in the future in ignorance or with secret vulgarised notions of sex physiology. The simple truth, told them little by little from the earliest age at which they begin to ask questions and in a way which will appeal to their idealism; then later teaching in the schools in biology, physiology, and nature study, will go far toward prevention, by introducing a new ideal. The teaching of older boys and girls should point to their responsibilities to future generations.

As a woman physician has well said, young men who might be deaf to the appeal of an individualistic morality may be moved to response by the presentation of their debt to race and country.

The education of fathers and mothers must, in the future, include the principles of heredity, the toxic effect of unholy passions upon temperament and character, and the study of eugenics, the new science for the improvement of the race of man.

First and last, women need to be encouraged to revolt against a status of political and legal inferiority which is the direct cause of their economic and social degradation.

PRACTICAL MEANS OF PREVENTION. These may be divided into two classes: one, the means of individual care or personal prevention of disease as such; the other, the means of social or deep-lying prevention of the *causes* of disease. The former is the more immediate, the latter more fundamental. The former will soon prove to be insufficient without the intervention of the latter. A comparison with other forms of infectious disease may serve as illustration.

When typhoid fever is epidemic, all persons are warned to boil their drinking water; yet Boards of Health are not satisfied with that individual precaution, but hold it necessary to protect remote sources of water supply, no matter how great the initial outlay of money.

In the warfare against tuberculosis, the first thing taught is the proper disposal of sputum, but no one rests satisfied with that, and presently it becomes evident that the whole question of housing and of occupation presses for solution, bringing with it the details of rent, of land monopoly, and of private ownership of the means of industry. Or, just as, in the expectation of raising a certain kind of crop, the farmer begins several years in advance by planting something quite different, or by expending capital on accessories, so must the social prevention of the social evil with its train of disease be arrived at by remote and indirect routes.

The personal precautions, being the most immediate, may be considered first.

PERSONAL PREVENTION OF VENEREAL DISEASE: CHILDHOOD. From earliest childhood there must be prevention of all habits known as self-abuse or masturbation, namely, all stimulation of the delicate nerve centres and fibres that are connected with the genital organs. Every nurse knows that such habits may arise even with babies, in complete innocence, of course, and that, if not checked, they may be less innocently continued by older children with grave danger both to health and morals. Mothers should be impressed with the dangers of this habit to the delicate and undeveloped nervous system of the child. Many do not know how real these dangers are, and regard the habit as an unimportant one, believing that it will be outgrown, as sometimes it may be. Nurses should teach the routine of absolute cleanliness of the parts, the avoidance of overwarm clothing, of idle luxurious living, of rich stimulating food, and above all, of alcoholic drinks for children, as all of these tend to excite the nervous system, while local irritants, such as uncleanliness or thick clumsy clothing, may act directly upon the nerves of the skin. Children should sleep in beds alone, with plenty of fresh air, and, if necessary to break up a tendency to self-handling, their hands should be so confined as to prevent tendency from becoming habit. Mothers should provide regular, skilled medical inspection for all children, that no abnormal condition may be overlooked. Sometimes such cases require surgical interference. The hygiene of the older child calls for ample physical and manual training, daily bathing with cool water, friction, and rough towels; regularity of all excretory functions; fresh air and not too much sedentary or solitary or monotonous occupation. In talking with mothers upon these subjects, nurses should have fortified themselves by careful instructions from the wisest medical men or women. Sensational prophecy of the possible results of masturbation may do great harm, yet negligence or timidity in controlling it may do even more. It is important that all mothers should understand that the younger the child is who forms the habit the more injurious is the practice in its effects upon the nervous system. Furthermore, it is the conviction of Dr. Morrow that masturbation tends to incline its victims toward immoral habits and leads young men to debauchery.

Dr. Blackwell, in her book, *The Human Element in Sex*, deals instructively with masturbation, specifying its chief evils as, 1, the injury to the mind through the nervous system, and, 2, the danger of habit-formation with resultant loss of self-control, with all the dangers that follow upon this loss of mastery over one's self, even to the destruction of health, insanity, or suicide. She says in another place: "Precocious physical development hinders moral development."

Löwenfeld, in discussing mental working power, says that it is oftener injured by masturbation than by excesses, adding:

and it is not always a case of very early or excessive masturbation; in many cases of this habit there are also painful reflections, such as self-reproach, self-accusation, anxiety for consequences, recollection of religious teachings, which affect the nervous system and through it the mental working power.

OLDER CHILDREN. For older children there should be definite warnings of the dangers which they may meet, as carefully and explicitly given as directions in taking a perilous journey. To leave little girls, especially, in ignorance of what these dangers are, is as wicked as it would be to expose them to wild beasts. Such warnings should be given at an early age. The little girl of twelve has a simple seriousness and sagacity, which may be looked for in vain if she remains untaught and undisciplined up to sixteen or seventeen, when youthful gaiety often runs into recklessness.

Such warnings need not cloud the happiness of childhood more than other necessary knowledge of danger which is likely to be met, and even if it does, better that than the tragic fate which now overtakes thousands of little girls. That kind of sentimentality which regards the ignorance of children in the face of the worst of perils as desirable and lovely, is a sickly and unsafe, it may be even a treacherous sentimentality. It would at least seem to be beyond contradiction that the age at which the laws cease giving protection to little girls should be the age at which they are to be armed with the knowledge which will help them to protect themselves.

YOUTH. Equally criminal is it to let the boys go to boarding-school or college without the most serious and intimate counsel and warnings against the horrible diseases lurking amidst the "wild oats" that they may thoughtlessly sow.

It is estimated by the records of the sickness insurance system of Germany that 25% of university students become infected with venereal diseases. We have no such statistics to guide us, but the writer has learned from the personal knowledge of the head of a large hospital in a great university centre, of the numbers of young men who come in for treatment for loathsome diseases. A painful feature of this calamity is that "the mothers are never told the truth; the fathers come and some reassuring falsehood is sent home." It is thus evident that, in such cases, the mere fact of the mother knowing the truth is greatly dreaded. Therefore, if it could be certain that all mothers would learn the truth, is it not likely that a powerful deterrent to evil courses in university life might be brought into play? If this is the result of silence and ignorance, the questions arise: "Is this really shielding the sanctity of home life? Are not these mothers guilty of a serious shirking of duty by not knowing, if their knowing would mean even partial prevention?"

EARLY ADULT LIFE. It is a hopeful sign that the ancient heresy of "physical necessity" for irregular indulgence by men, so long upheld by them, tacitly assented to by women, and even sometimes taught by high medical authorities, is now being gradually repudiated and denied by the most eminent physicians and hygienists. To maintain it has been, indeed, an insult to all those men whose lives are and have been pure, and one must wonder that such men have so long permitted so detestable a doctrine to go unchallenged. Young men may now be taught, with all the authority of science, that the same virtue which is desirable for their sisters is good for them, and that "physical necessity," like drug habits, only grows coarser and ranker by indulgence and weakening of the will power. Self-control is an evidence of a strong and manly nature and of a well-balanced physical endowment.

MARRIAGE. Medical statistics show that the vast majority of all innocently contracted cases of venereal disease are those contracted by wives and children through the institution of marriage: that fifty per cent. of the sterility of wives and from twenty to twenty-five per cent. of the sterility of husbands is caused by the *gonococcus:* that a large per cent. of miscarriages and a heavy infant mortality are due to the *Spirochæte pallida:* that fully eighty per cent. of blindness from birth and twenty-five per cent. of all blindness is gonorrhœal: that the secondary symptoms of inherited syphilis often cause loss of sight or hearing: that from fifty to seventy-five per cent. of all gynecological operations, often involving amputation of the female organs of generation, and an indefinite proportion of all cases of chronic, life-long invalidism in women result from the deadly power of persistence of the *gonococcus* and its tendency to remain latent in the male organs, suddenly to kindle an acute inflammation in the virgin tissues to which it may gain access: it is therefore plain that the most extreme precautions of personal prevention need to be taken before the risk of marriage is run. No parent should allow a daughter to marry without securing authentic proof that the promised husband is free from disease. This is incontestably a duty of parents of the utmost gravity and importance, neglecting which all their previous care, expense, and nurture lavished on the daughter may go for naught. An honourable and virtuous man will willingly give such testimony, and might rightly demand on his side assurances from the parents as to their daughter's inheritance. Such inquiries are not impossible. They could all be conducted by the trusted physicians of one or both families with entire privacy and dignity. Fathers find ways to inform themselves of the business standing of prospective sons-in-law, and health is far more precious than money.

What personal prevention can there be for an innocent partner in marriage, if in later years infection is brought to her from prostitution? It would seem that here, as in the case of the college boy, the knowledge that the truth would surely become known might in many cases act as a deterrent. At present the victim (usually the wife) is kept in ignorance of the real cause of her illness. Certainly, if there is any inalienable right of the individual, it is to know what is the matter with one when one is ill. But at present two barriers are interposed: one is the general ignorance of the laity in matters of health preservation; the other is medical reticence. Only when women have sufficient general knowledge of health and disease, and courage to insist on the truth and to accept it when offered, can the second barrier be broken down. Already many physicians are chafing against the shackles of the "medical secret," and they are sometimes severely blamed for their share in the general blindfolding of the public in regard to venereal diseases. Yet to speak the truth in individual cases exposes them to suits-at-law and other most trying experiences. It can, however, hardly be doubted that the certainty of truth being known would in time have a salutary preventive effect upon married men. It would at least be a simple justice to their victims.

PREVENTION OF ACCIDENTAL INFECTION. Remembering the characteristics of the *Spirochæte pallida*, its extreme virulence while living, but short life period outside the body; and those of the *gonococcus*, with its equal or even greater virulence and perhaps somewhat greater tenacity of life outside the body; remembering that neither is conveyed by dust or through the air, but only by material objects, it should be possible for every one to guard against accidental infection, without suffering from exaggerated alarm. Common drinking cups, as in railway cars and public places, should be absolutely avoided. Individuals should carry their own cups. Progressive railroads are now providing individual drinking cups of paper, to be used once and then thrown away. They should be demanded of every public service corporation. Towels, too, in common use, must always be regarded as possible carriers. They should never be applied to the face and 'eyes unless freshly laundered. In general, it should be a matter of universal practice never to rub or even touch the eyes except with a clean piece of linen—never with the fingers or finger nails, as they carry all manner of infectious germs.

The face should not be washed directly from basins that are used indiscriminately, especially for rinsing the mouth. Rubbing the face with a clean wet towel may be substituted in travelling.

Eating utensils which have been washed and dried may be regarded as probably safe, yet in many places it would no doubt be an added security to carry one's own fork and spoon. The fresh cleanliness of bed linen cannot be too carefully looked into when travelling. The conditions of public laundries should also be a matter of investigation by housekeepers. The seats of public water-closets may always be regarded as being more or less doubtful, and when used, may be covered with a clean piece of paper. Many cases of gonorrhœa are caused by the dirty or ill-kept seats of public conveniences, especially in crowded places. Public bath tubs should be used with precautions of thorough cleansing, and if doubtful, had better be let alone. No object should ever be put to the lips or eyes which may have been so handled by other persons, such as pencils, pens, sticks, etc. To put money into the mouth should be forbidden by the Boards of Health. The importance of having individual towels, face-cloths, napkins, utensils, etc., is now generally recognised in institutions, homes, asylums, and schools. Such articles are, if used in common, of course capable of conveying many kinds of infection, and it will be seen that the avoidance of mechanical contagion of venereal disease is much like that of tuberculosis and pus diseases, the chief difference being that of the absence of danger from dust in the one and its great danger in the others.

In caring for cases of venereal diseases, nurses and others should observe as rigid a technic of disinfection as in diphtheria or other acute infectious fevers. All discharges from the mucous membranes, ulcerated or suppurating tissues, eyes, mouth, or nose should be received on clean waste material and promptly burned. Clothing and bed linen should be boiled or sterilised, then well sunned and aired. The danger of infecting laundresses by unsterilised clothing should always be remembered. Complete isolation of dishes and utensils should be observed and they should be periodically boiled. Patients with mucous patches should never expectorate carelessly, for, though the dried germs are not dangerous, there is always the possibility of direct contact in some manner before the death of the germs. Nor should such patients sneeze or cough without carefully protecting their surroundings by covering the nose or mouth. This, indeed, should be the usual routine for all persons at all times.

It is the right of every nurse, for self-protection, to know what she is taking care of, and it should be impressed upon all nurses that they must invariably insist upon knowing the diagnosis in the cases they care for. It has not infrequently happened that nurses, kept by the attending physician in ignorance of the venereal origin of patients' maladies, have contracted them. It is also true that if all nurses were sufficiently well taught and trained, it should be second nature with them to avoid all infectious contact. The proper precautions being observed, nurses and all others should comprehend clearly that there is no danger whatever from the simple presence of cases of venereal disease amidst other people, and no more danger in caring for them than there is with cases of ordinary sepsis. Accidental infection arises solely from ignorance; this cannot be too strongly emphasised. Proof is amply given by the results of well-managed venereal wards, where infection of attendants and nurses does not occur. French experts have recently recommended the inclusion of adult venereal patients (with the possible exception of extreme cases) in the general wards of hospitals for the sake of the better moral and mental influence, and explain that the recommendation is perfectly practicable because with the proper technic of care such patients need not be regarded as dangerous from the stand-point of infection.

In conclusion it should be remembered that there are probably no other diseases where early and competent medical advice is more all-important. If quackery is always a blunder, here it is a fatal one, and nurses should use their whole power as teachers to impress this on their communities. All the social circumstances connected with the time of cure and return of such patients to normal life make the necessity for the best medical oversight one of paramount importance.

SOCIAL PREVENTION OF PROSTITUTION. In order to approach social methods of preventing prostitution in a perfectly intelligent way there should first be three main lines of inquiry, which can here be simply indicated, in the briefest fashion, as lines on which there is work waiting for women to do. They are:

First, to discover the extent of prostitution. Second, to ascertain its various reasons for existence,—what they are and how much diversity they have to show. Third, to penetrate to the social arrangements in which these reasons are imbedded, and to see how much there is here that is artificial and needless.

The right attitude of mind with which to undertake such inquiry is, that it is rational to believe that prostitution and its resultant diseases can be reduced to a minimum, and that it is possible for that minimum to be discovered. To be convinced that it can be and inflexibly determined that it must be discovered is no more visionary or theoretical than it has been in the past to believe in all the dawning possibilities of human progress. There was a time when it was thought that the plague, typhus, smallpox, and other infectious diseases could not be conquered.

Science has indeed not banished any of these ills entirely from the earth, but it has given society the knowledge of how to keep them down to their lowest terms.

THE EXTENT OF PROSTITUTION. It is doubtful whether correct figures could be obtained at present of the entire extent of prostitution. This would be the first task to undertake in initiating an aggressive campaign against the institution as such. But, taking the world over, being guided by the statements that are made by officials and social students regarding single cities and countries, it is hardly doubtful that there are, in all, several million women set aside in this life. It was stated at the Brussels congress, conservatively, that there were fifty thousand in England. Taber Johnson estimates the number in the United States at about half a million who are in houses of ill-fame, and believes there may be as many more outside of such places. In exerting the imagination to picture this number of women pariahs and to call them together in one mass before the mental vision in order to personify them, and to consider the problem of their relation to disease, it is to be remembered that this dreary race does not perpetuate itself. Prostitutes quickly become sterile, and few leave children. Their lives, moreover, are very short. Some authorities estimate the average life of the prostitute as ten years; some believe it to be even less,—a five-year average. Between these two estimates it may be possible there is a mean, but even this is sufficiently short, especially as it does not signify their working life, so to speak, but the actual span of life. In from five to ten years they die, many from pneumonia, tuberculosis, alcoholism, and suicide, while practically all of them, says Dr. Morrow, finally become cases of venereal disease of one form or another. Now, if it were only this half-million or so of women in our own country who were doomed to early disease and premature death for no better or more useful reason than to gratify the brutal and selfish lusts of men that will finally destroy those very men themselves, this alone would be a disgrace to modern hygiene and civilisation. It may be illustrated by supposing that a half-million women were set apart at any one time in our great country to be infected with leprosy or to be compelled to die of diphtheria. All the health boards of the country would be in a state of desperate activity, and the daily press would find no headlines sufficiently sensational. But it is actually even worse than this, for, in order to fill the vacancies caused by disease and death, some 50,000 fresh and once at least pure, clean, and innocent young girls must be annually drafted into this death-dealing business.

Solely as a matter of public health, without regarding moral considerations for a moment, this is a danger of paramount importance, yet it meets with less concern from health boards than half-a-dozen smallpox cases. Indeed, the discovery of one smallpox case is telegraphed all over the country, but the fact that numbers of young girls are set aside yearly to die of venereal disorders and their tragic accompaniments is ignored by sanitary departments and the press.

From this point of view, too, the extent of prostitution as the source of venereal disease must be noted in the light of the computation of experts, that for every abandoned woman there are at the least five profligate men. Dr. Morrow estimates, from carefully collected data, that, of the young men in this country reaching their sixteenth year (numbering 770,000 annually), at least sixty per cent. or over 450,000 of each year's cohort, will, at some time of life, become infected with venereal disease, and that twenty per cent. of such infection will occur before the end of the twenty-first year.

REASONS FOR THE EXISTENCE OF PROSTITUTION. What are these reasons and how diverse are they? The statements of the United States District-Attorney, as well as of speakers at the Brussels conferences, indicating that about four fifths of all prostitutes are unwillingly such, though painful, have a hopeful aspect, as they point definitely to the conclusion that prostitution is capable of being reduced to an easily controllable minimum. If these four fifths of unwilling members of the sad army could be withheld from entering this life, it would not be an insoluble problem to deal with the remaining fifth. Distributed, as they would be, over the whole country, the number of "chronic or persevering" prostitutes with which each community had to deal would not be an unmanageable number. If they were irreclaimable, they could be kept in colonies, tenderly and wisely cared for, as are the insane and feeble-minded. If this ideal method should be too advanced, then, when there were really only the prostitutes by preference to consider, and then only, might direct legislation of a punitive character for women be spoken of without bitter injustice and wrong.

The only true prevention for such chronic or determined evil-doers, and the prevention that the future must show how to apply, is, not to have them born. Who can say, now, that they are not the inevitable hereditary consequences of their parents' sexual excesses?

Unwilling victims of a stupid social order should not be regarded as true prostitutes, but as sacrifices, as human loss and waste due to pure mismanagement. The underlying reason for their lapse is poverty or the unequal struggle against want. All medical and social experts who have studied this problem agree that prostitution is a disease of poverty. Testimony on this point is so abundant that it is not necessary to prove the point here, but it may be recalled that the favourite buttress for the arguments of those who uphold prostitution and licensed vice is the dictum that "there must always be prostitution because there will always be poverty."

Poverty, then, must be so far eradicated or at least so far mitigated that it cannot honestly be given as an explanation of prostitution. This is the social prevention of venereal diseases which are fostered in prostitution.

It will now be clear how far-reaching and remote are the paths along which the prevention of venereal diseases must be pursued. They lead even farther than the road to the prevention of typhoid fever, which follows the water-courses back to the pure springs of the head-waters. And they are obstructed by the same obstacles in the mercenary interests that have become parasitic; but besides all these they are blocked by one obstacle which no other contagious disease has ever had to meet, namely, the selfish and hitherto uncontrolled pleasure of indulgence of the individual man. The prevalence and power of this pleasure-lust make it hopeless to expect that a majority of men will give it up themselves of their own volition; and vain, therefore, is it to look to their management for prevention of prostitution. It will be found again, as Mrs. Butler found, that many will readily lop off the worst manifestations of this institution, such as the white slave traffic, who will never whole-heartedly undertake the eradication of the institution itself. Already this is clear in the articles which are now appearing in the periodicals and daily papers upon the white slave trade; horror of the trade is freely expressed, with shame and contrition for its existence, but one may search vainly through the lay press for any bugle-call to men to put an end to prostitution. This must be the work of women, and to do it they must possess the instrument which is as indispensable in controlling the acts of legislatures, which lie behind all social conditions, as is the microscope to the physician in his research work, or the scissors to the mother who is cutting out her children's clothes.

ENFRANCHISEMENT OF WOMEN THE FIRST STEP. Long ago Dr. Taylor said that every method had been tried for the prevention of venereal disease except one, and that was the teaching of continence to young men. But Dr. Taylor was wrong, though a good and noble man; for in his day no one had ever dreamed of trying the remedy of giving power and authority to the mothers of young men. And it is passing strange that so few even of the men sincerely desirous of wiping these scourges of disease from the earth should think of this remedy, even when, as at the Brussels conferences, they have racked their brains for suggestions and have put forth some that seem almost childish in their grasping at straws. For now it is possible to see the beginnings of what women will do with this matter of prostitution and venereal disease when they have full political power. To-day, the only parts of the world where this combined problem is progressing toward solution are those parts where women have been in possession of the ballot long enough to show some results of their direct influence.[1]

Only the determination of women who are politically free, expressed through the machinery of government by the right use of popular government's only instrument, the ballot, can effect the downfall of prostitution as a social and commercial institution. Some broad-minded men there are who do see this. Professor James Stuart said to Miss Emily Ford, of England, when she asked what could be done to stop commercialised vice, *"Go on trying for woman suffrage"*; while in our own country there are medical members of the American Society of Sanitary and Moral Prophylaxis who take the same position.

SOCIAL STEPS IN PREVENTION. There must be

[1] See Appendix B.

full and ample protection for children from the very cradle,—yes, even earlier. It must be possible for every child to be well-born, and the pregnant mother must be protected first from want, poverty, and sweated labour.

Child labour must be abolished and child-culture substituted for it. Children that are forced into the labour market are almost foredoomed to prostitution and venereal disease because their enfeeblement and premature exhaustion weakens will power, retards useful education, and warps their natures, whilst the exposure to all sorts of moral dangers cannot be avoided by little wage-slaves. The need of ample legal protection for little girls has been sufficiently shown by the facts of the "age of consent" laws. These laws and the resistance of legislatures to their amendment, show only too plainly that they have been intentionally framed and kept, not for the protection of girls, but for the protection of men while keeping an open door through which a sufficient supply of young girls may be continually passed into ruin. This is a painful reflection, but it is the only possible conclusion from the facts.

But further, for the real protection of girls not only legislation, but vigilant administration and unswerving enforcement of law must be had. Now, the former, or some appearance of it, may indeed be secured as a concession from men, but the latter can never be hoped for until women possess the same public and legal powers that men now possess.[1] This is a point that is almost invariably overlooked. The flippant query so often heard, "Shall we have women police?" needs to be answered seriously in the affirmative; women are urgently, desperately needed as police wherever young children and growing creatures are out in the world, and the time may not be far off when such police, with the training of the nurse or the teacher, shall be more numerous than those we are now familiar with. Then, and for the first time, there will be real "morals police." Widowed mothers must not be compelled to act as father and mother both, by being driven to earn their children's bread outside the home while trying to keep their little ones in the home. Through this double burden women have been driven to the streets, or their little ones have found the way there. There are seas of sentimentality poured forth about the home,—but it never seems to be the home of the working people

[1] See Appendix C.

that is meant. Yet these are the majority of the homes. To one of America's deepest-hearted and most clear-seeing women, a sight that seemed too intolerable to be borne was the sight of a working mother whose abundant milk dripped to the floor as she scrubbed business offices for sixteen hours a day. Who can tell how such sins against family life will end?

The real protection of mothers and of children will be, as to prostitution and venereal disease, what the protection of the head-waters is to typhoid fever; for, as Judge Lindsay's recent true story has shown, *it is absolutely essential for the children to be ruined at a tender age, if a vicious and corrupt class is to be maintained.*[1]

The fundamental and crying need in the protection of older girls is a living wage. It is only too well known that employers in every country where women are disfranchised have not infrequently given to their young employees, along with their wage pittances, the suggestion that it is always open to them to earn more without difficulty. The researches recently made by the National Consumers' League into the relation between the cost of living and the wages paid

[1] See Appendix D.

to girls in industry in New York City, striking as they have been in their demonstration of gross inequality, give cause for added thought in view of the official information that that city is the centre of the white slave trade.[1]

Hours of work need to be shortened for all workers. Overwork, monotony, and chronic fatigue make all work hateful and destroy healthful ideals, while the long hours of work leave no time for natural enjoyment or pleasure in life.

It is often said, as a piece of superior wisdom, that men cannot be made moral by law. It is only superficially true. Conditions which make young boys and girls, young women and men, or older women and men immoral by necessity can be and should be altered by the law. Indeed they must be, because the whole modern social structure rests finally on the support given to it by laws. Intelligent social legislation, when rightly enforced, is like the fence that keeps marauders out of an orchard. Vainly does the gardener put forth his best work if the fence is not there and the despoilers are. If we could get rid of marauders, we might do without fences, as the French gardens need none.

[1] See Appendix E.

The influence of unenfranchised women is nullified and frustrated precisely as are the efforts of the unprotected gardener. Her fence will be the ballot, but she must build it herself. The marauders who threaten her are all the vicious and dangerous elements among men who know that her supremacy means the ultimate disappearance of that social evil on which they base all their profitable exploitation of the young and the helpless. These enemies, though the most venomous, are the most silent; they are never heard in arguments against woman suffrage.[1]

English women writers, medical women and the leaders of the suffrage movement both in England and in our own country, declare in the most explicit terms that the real hostility to the advance of women comes from those who exploit prostitution, while, on the other hand, at the foundation of the terrible earnestness of the women of England to gain the Parliamentary franchise is the burning and unflinching determination to free womanhood from this disgrace. In this country the story is the same, though not so well understood by the great mass of women.

The fear of the "bad woman's vote" has long

[1] See Appendix F.

been dangled as a spectre before the eyes of timid good women. How fictitious this fear is may be realised by summing up the testimony proving that eighty per cent. of the "bad women" need not have been bad; that almost all prostitution is commercial, and that its promoters rely chiefly for their supplies on the ruin of children of tender years, eking out with young girls snared in their silly and thoughtless age; that the white slave trade is now and always has been supported and protected by men politically corrupt; that in Colorado, where all women vote, the "bad women" actually cast just one third of one per cent. of the vote of Denver[1]; that the women of that State, though in the minority, have succeeded in placing model statutes for the protection and training of children upon the books, and have helped to maintain in power against bitter enemies the one man fearless enough to enforce and reinforce them, while in the three other enfranchised states not a word is ever heard about a "bad" vote; that in New Zealand prostitution has been reduced to its lowest terms, while commercialised vice is practically extinct there. Well did Dr.

[1] Dr. Aylesworth, in his Carnegie Hall address, Nov. 17, 1909.

Aylesworth say, "These women [the prostitutes] exert a hundred fold more influence upon politicians through their business than through their ballots."

A New Ideal Needed. A new ideal needs to be formed; an ideal of the worth and dignity of human life, and of a commanding place and power that must be assumed by women in all that pertains to the cherishing and ennobling of the race. This ideal must be built upon the single standard of sex morality and it must be attained by a gradual process of assumption of knowledge and authority by women, to the end that they may finally produce a nobler and a finer race of men.

SOURCES OF MATERIAL USED IN THE PREPARATION OF PART III.

Abbott, Edith, Women in Industry. 1909.
American Society of Sanitary and Moral Prophylaxis. Publications. 9 East 42d St., New York City.
    The Boy Problem: For Parents and Teachers.
    The Young Man's Problems: For Teachers.
    The Relations of Social Diseases with Marriage, and their Prophylaxis.
    How My Uncle, the Doctor, Instructed Me in Matters of Sex.
    Health and the Hygiene of Sex: for College Students.
Anthony, Susan B., and Harper, Ida Husted, History of Woman Suffrage. 4 vols.
Arendt, Sister Henriette (for five years assistant police officer in Stuttgart, in charge of women prisoners before and after their discharge), Menschen die den Pfad Verloren. Stuttgart, 1907.
Aves, Ernest, Report to the Secretary of State for the Home Department on the Wages Boards and Industrial Conciliation and Arbitration Acts of Australia and New Zealand. London, 1908. (Blue Book.)
Blackwell, Elizabeth, M.D., Counsel to Parents on the Moral Education of Their Children. 1880.
Blackwell, Elizabeth, M.D., The Human Element in Sex, 1884.
Blackwell, Elizabeth, M.D., The Laws of Life, with Special Reference to the Physical Education of Girls. 1852.
Blackwell, Elizabeth, M.D., Medicine and Morality.
Blackwell, Elizabeth, M.D., Pioneer Work in Opening the Medical Profession to Women. 1896.

Blackwell, Elizabeth, M.D., The Religion of Health.
Blackwell, Elizabeth, M.D., Wrong and Right Methods of Dealing with Social Evil. (No date; about 1860-70.)
Broadhead, State Regulation of Labour and Labour Disputes in New Zealand. 1908.
Bureau of Labour, Labour Conditions in Australia (Bulletin, Vol. X., 1905).
Bureau of Labour, Minimum Wages Act of 1908 in New South Wales, p. 86. (Bulletin No. 80. January, 1909.)
Conference on the Care of Dependent Children, Washington, D. C., January 25, 26, 1909. Proceedings.
Eugenics Education Society. Publications. London.
Immigration Committee, Report. Importing Women for Immoral Purposes. (Senate Document No. 196.)
Jacobi, Mary Putnam, M.D., Common-Sense Applied to Woman Suffrage. New York, 1894.
Kelley, Florence, Some Ethical Gains Through Legislation. New York, 1905.
Löwenfeld, Die geistige Arbeitskraft. In Grenzfragen des Nerven und Seelenlebens. Vol. vi.
Macrosty, State Arbitration and the Minimum Wage in Australasia. In Trade Unionism and Labour Problems, edited with an Introduction by John R. Commons, p. 195. New York, 1905.
Martindale, L., M.D., Under the Surface. Brighton, England.
National American Woman Suffrage Association. Political Equality Leaflets:
    Blackwell, Alice Stone, Fruits of Equal Suffrage, i., ii.
    Holder, Lady, Equal Suffrage in Australia.
    Kelley, Florence, Woman Suffrage: Its Relation to Working Women and Children.
    Macnaghten, R. E., Women's Vote in Australia.
    Nathan, Maud, Wage Earner and the Ballot.
    Russell, Charles Edward, Woman Suffrage in New Zealand.
    Wells, Mrs. Borrman, New Zealand's Experience.
New York Probation Association. First Report. 165 W. 10th St., New York City.

Sources of Material Used

Oregon and Illinois Briefs relating to Overwork. The Consumers' League, 105 E. 22d St., New York City.
Roosevelt's (President) Homes Commission Report. (Senate Document No. 644.)
Royal Commission on the Poor Laws. Minority Report. London, 1909.
University of London, Eugenics Laboratory Lecture Series. London.

APPENDIX A

ATTEMPTS TO INTRODUCE REGULATION INTO THE UNITED STATES

St. Louis: Attempt made in 1870 under pretext of suppressing prostitution. The words "or regulate" introduced into a clause of the city charter established a system of supervised vice which continued until 1874, when it was abolished by the force of public indignation.

California: In 1871 the legislature had a bill brought before it for legalising and regulating vice. The wife of a member drew up and had presented a bill identical with the first except that the word "man" was substituted throughout where the word "woman" appeared in the original bill. The obnoxious bill was withdrawn.

Cincinnati: In 1874 an attempt was made to regulate vice by enactment but it was defeated.

Pennsylvania: In 1874 a bill was presented in the legislature for the State regulation of vice. Fifty-two medical men sent a noble protest, affirming the single moral standard. The bill was defeated.

DISTRICT OF COLUMBIA: Regulation by the Board of Health was proposed in 1875 and was defeated.

NEW YORK STATE: About the same date similar legislation brought before the legislature was defeated by the power of Elizabeth Cady Stanton, Susan B. Anthony, and their allies.

[Data taken from *A Comparative Survey of Laws*, etc., by Sheldon Amos.]

APPENDIX B

EXAMPLES OF THE KIND OF LEGISLATION WOMEN ARE ESPECIALLY INTERESTED IN AND WORK FOR

WYOMING: Equal pay to men and women teachers of equal qualification.

Age of protection for girls raised to 18.

Penalties for neglect, abuse, or cruelty shown to children.

Prohibition of the labour of boys under 14 in mines.

No cigarettes, liquor, or tobacco to be sold or given to persons under 16.

Free public kindergartens established.

Licensed gambling forbidden.

Provision for the care and custody of deserted or orphan children and children of infirm, indigent, or incompetent persons.

COLORADO: State home for dependent children established. Two of the five members of the board of managers must be women.

Provision that at least three out of six members of the board of county visitors shall be women.

Mothers made joint guardians of their children with the fathers [this equality of parents exists in only thirteen of the States of the Union].

Age of protection for girls raised to 18.

State industrial home for girls established; three of the five members of the board of managers to be women.

Protective care for the feeble-minded provided.

Woman physician placed on the board of the asylums for the insane.

Juvenile courts and truant schools established; education compulsory to the 16th year.

Union high schools established.

Advanced regulations for child labour and an eight-hour day for children of 16 or under.

Prohibition for over eight hours a day for women working in occupations that require standing.

To contribute to the delinquency of a child made a criminal offence.

IDAHO: Gambling made illegal.

Age of protection for girls raised to 18.

Industrial reform school established.

Equalisation of married women's rights in property.

UTAH: Equal pay for men and women teachers equally qualified.

Age of protection for girls raised to 18.

Sale or gift of cigarettes, tobacco, opium, or any other narcotic to persons under 18 forbidden.

Provisions for protection of children against neglect or ill treatment.

Free kindergartens established.

[The above examples have been taken from pamphlets by Alice Stone Blackwell: *Fruits of Equal Suffrage*, I. and II. Only those that are specially pertinent to the subject under discussion in the text have been chosen, whilst the pamphlets themselves give numerous other examples without assuming to show a complete list. It is pointed out that laws of this character are much better enforced where women are enfranchised. The leaflets are published by the National American Woman Suffrage Association, 505 Fifth Avenue, New York City.]

NEW ZEALAND: Legal standard of morality and conditions of divorce made the same for men and women.

Legal separation from worthless husbands obtainable summarily and without expense.

Testator's Family Maintenance Act prevents a man from willing away his property without making suitable provision for wife and family.

Old-age pensions for aged persons... old couple may receive a joint pension... home.

Government asylums for inebriates...

Health of women workers and of workers of both sexes under 18 carefully protected; hours of labour and legal holidays with payment regulated (the eight-hour day is legal]; payment of wages to workmen in trades secured and workers' compensation for accidents defined with great advantage to the working people.

Purer code of morals established by alterations in the criminal code.

Adoption of children regulated by law and baby farming prevented.

Industrial schools and technical schools established.

[From *Woman Suffrage in New Zealand*, published by the International Woman Suffrage Alliance. Leaflet No. 1.]

AUSTRALIA: On the federal domain the chief gains so far are:

Equal pay for equal work in government departments.

Naturalisation laws made equal for men and women.

Unified marriage and divorce bills.

In the separate (Australian) states the gains are: wages boards; children's courts; old-age pensions; protection for wage-earning children; married women's property acts; aid for the illegitimate mother; reforms in the drink trade.

[From *Where Women have the Vote*, published by the National Union of Women's Suffrage Societies, 25 Victoria St., Westminster, London; quoting Miss Alice Zimmern's *Women's Suffrage in Many Lands*.]

APPENDIX C

SOME STATISTICS OF CRIMINAL ASSAULT UPON YOUNG GIRLS [1]

By Mary Burr, Delegate to the International Congress of Nurses of the National Council of Trained Nurses of Great Britain and Ireland.

Statistics are usually considered very dry, but when those figures mean ruined lives, as they do in this paper, then they assume an aspect which should command our very closest attention. In endeavouring to gather these statistics, it was originally intended to draw as far as possible upon private sources. These, however, proved inadequate, and a dozen different societies which deal with wronged women and children were approached for whatever information they could give.

The results proved somewhat curious; from only

[1] Read at the International Congress of Nurses, London, July, 1909. Reprinted in the *British Journal of Nursing*, Nov. 6, 1909.

two did I receive any definite information—the National Society for the Prevention of Cruelty to Children and the Church Penitentiary Association.

Of the other societies, six referred me to some one else, and even the National Vigilance Society, from which I expected much, referred me to the Director of Public Prosecutions; the remainder said they did not deal with such cases.

One lady flatly refused to furnish information which she considered private to a congress of which she knew nothing.

It made one wonder if this work, which so closely affects the national well-being, is a private preserve, reserved to those who work in it. It almost appears so. Information was sought on four points only:

1. The number of cases of criminal assault committed upon young girls and children.
2. The number of cases in which prosecution followed.
3. The result of the prosecution.
4. The ages of the victims.

The idea was to find out as far as possible the extent of this awful evil; what proportion of the offenders were punished and the degree of punishment inflicted, because, of various cases which had come to my knowledge, only a very small proportion were brought to justice. As so little information was obtained from the societies from which I had hoped to gain so much, I took the advice of one secretary, and bought the Blue Book of Criminal Statistics, and here is the result.

Comparative statistics are given for 15 years from 1893 to 1907; the details of 1907 only are given. In those 15 years there were 2302 cases of defilement of girls under 13 years of age, and 2442 cases of defilement of girls under 16 years of age, making the terrible total of 4744 cases reported to the police.

Of these 3425 were tried—1660 for assault on girls under 13, the remaining 1765 being for girls under 16.

The details of the cases for 1907, which are included in the above figures, are as follows:—Reported to the police, 149 cases concerning girls under 13, and 178 concerning girls under 16; total, 327. Of these, 97 of the first and 135 of the latter were tried, a total of 232 cases, roughly about two thirds. Five cases were thrown out, 82 were acquitted, 145 convicted. The punishment of those convicted was penal servitude in 23 cases for terms varying from four to twenty years, five and seven years being the usual sentence; one man was flogged; the remainder received terms of imprisonment from fourteen days to two years.

One curious fact in this grim document is the distinction drawn between girls under and over 13.

All the sentences of penal servitude were given in the former cases, and not one in the latter; apparently a girl over 13 and under 16 may be treated in the most dastardly manner and the sentence be anything between fourteen days and two years.

This does not conclude the terrible sum of immorality among the males of this Christian land, for during the years quoted—1893 to 1907—there were also 3407 cases of rape, and 12,280 cases of indecent assault upon women over 16, reported to the police, altogether making the ghastly total of 15,687 cases reported, and with the 4744 cases under 16, we have the tremendous number of 20,431—an annual average for the fifteen years of 1362 women's lives wrecked. Such is the information from the Blue Book.

The Rev. Thomas George Cree, Hon. Secretary of the Church Penitentiary Association, sent me a very interesting little pamphlet, *Juvenile Immorality*, in which he states that he sent out a circular to all the homes and refuges on their list asking for the number of such children under 16 dealt with during the last three years (up to October, 1908). Replies from 40 penitentiaries were received; 7 did not take such cases, the 33 which did returned 347 cases. From 55 refuges the number of cases returned was 745; total for three years, 1092.

Some of the details are as follows:—8 cases between 6 and 8 years of age; 18 between 9 and 11 years; 11 cases of 12 years; 14 cases of 13 years; 121 cases of 14 years; and 301 cases of 15 years.

In one town the Chief Constable reports that hardly a child over 14 years has not fallen. From another, that children under 14 absolutely solicit in considerable numbers. In another, lads marked with badges solicit. On inquiring why prosecutions are so few, the reply comes from all quarters that so often the culprit is the father, step-father, uncle, or brother of the victim. In a covering letter, Mr. Cree writes that, besides the numbers already quoted, fully 1000 more cases were known, but the parents would not allow the rescue workers to deal with them.

He says convictions are *very* few, as relations are often the culprits, and prosecutions must be taken in hand within six months after the commission of the crime; and, when there is danger of an infant being born, the child is restrained by threats from saying anything until its state is manifest.

Also young children are subject to cross-examination by lawyers, and he states a case of a child of 10 being cross-examined for a full hour, but the evidence could not be shaken, and the case was sent to the Assizes.

From the Society for the Prevention of Cruelty

to Children came the statistics for last year—838 cases, 146 prosecuted, 46 being dismissed.

Of collected cases there are 20, 18 of these being under 16, one being only 3 and another 5 years of age. In two the fathers were the culprits, and in one the brother was suspected. In six of these cases nothing was done, either because parents would not prosecute, or for want of sufficient evidence. Two of these cases were very bad. One, a girl, went to a gardener's for fruit at midday on Sunday, did not return home until 6.30; then went out, presumably to chapel. Nothing more was seen of her until her body was taken from the river on the following Tuesday morning. On examination, the child was found to have been violated. The gardener was severely censured at the inquest, and an open verdict given.

The other was of a child of 12, who was outraged while her mother was lying dead. The child accused her father of the crime, but, as it could not be proved, he was let off.

Out of 11 cases which were investigated, 3 were discharged, 1 because there was, as the Judge said, "No corroboration," and 1 "not proven." Of the 6 convicted, 1 was let off with a fine, and the others received sentences varying from six months to ten years.

Of the two cases over 16, one was a girl of 17

mentally deficient, and the culprits (several youths, one of whom confessed to the wrong-doing) were all discharged by the magistrates. The other, also a girl of 17, was seized from behind, a drugged handkerchief stuffed into her mouth, and she was dragged into the bracken off the high road across a Surrey heath. There she was outraged, and when she recognised her assailant, he tried to pour poison down her throat, fortunately without much success. Chiefly because of the attempt to poison he got seven years. I think it should have been for life.

If such is the condition of things as they are known, what number of cases are there unknown? If there are 327 cases *reported* during a year, how very many hundreds are there unreported? Yet men who are supposed to protect the weak take every advantage of that weakness. Governments come and go, yet this terrible evil remains unchecked. Why have not these cases been put in the same category as murder? Do our law-makers consider it worse to kill the body than to outrage its honour and sully its soul?

It is useless to try, as some may do, to blame foreigners; only one culprit among all the reported cases for 1907 was an alien.

These men, who defile women and violate their own offspring, are British. They have the power of helping to make the laws which we women must obey, and, judging from these statistics, make them as easy as possible for the indulgence of their own lusts.

If this is not so, why must cases be instituted within six months of the offence? Why must a child, whose whole moral and physical nature has been so recently outraged, be subjected to cross-examination by a lawyer (a man) upon so delicate a matter?

And, lastly, how is it possible to expect corroborative evidence in the majority of such cases?

If such a state of things is the result of the absolute political power of men, the sooner women have votes the better it will be for the nation, and the sooner will its moral and physical condition be improved.

INADEQUATE PROTECTION TO GIRLS

" A sinister chapter to which too little attention has hitherto been paid is the failure of our legislatures and courts to afford to young girls protection from seduction, assault, and enslavement in infamous houses. The difficulty involved in obtaining the conviction of malefactors is known only to the few faithful souls who have attempted to obtain due punishment of these grave offences. Mothers in any community are more deeply stirred by these offences than by any others, but judges and juries vary beyond belief in their ... of crimes against girls.

"In one western State a woman worked ... years to obtain the enactment of a ... to punish crimes against females, ... such a law was passed and vigorously ... teen criminals were sent to the penitentiary. Then a young lawyer offered his services to one of the criminals, to free him by showing that the law was unconstitutional because the title should have read: '*to define and* punish crimes against female minors' whereas in fact the two words '*define and*' were missing from the title, though the necessary definition was contained in the body of the statute. Upon this frivolous ground the Supreme court of the State held the statute invalid, and nine of the fourteen criminals were forthwith freed. The others were too poor or too ignorant to obtain counsel, and they remained in the penitentiary."[1]

EXAMPLES OF LAWMAKING IN NEW YORK STATE

The maximum punishment that can be given to a "cadet," or man	Section 1566 of the penal code of New York State, which is conspicu-

[1] *Woman Suffrage: its Relation to Working Women and Children*, by Florence Kelley, published by the National American Woman Suffrage Association.

who lives upon the earnings of prostitutes, in New York State is six months in the workhouse. The statute makes this offence a misdemeanour.

ously placed in the surface cars fixes one year's imprisonment and $500 fine as the maximum penalty for stealing or giving away a transfer ticket worth five cents.

The offence of "procuring" is graver, and is punishable with the same degree of severity as is the offence of spitting on the floors of cars and public buildings.

APPENDIX D

PROTECTION OF WIDOWED MOTHERS

The possibilities of protection extended by the state to mothers with children who are dependent on them, not only for care but for a livelihood, are indicated by the systems of industrial insurance or compensation now in force in almost every civilised country except this one. Every European country, at the present time, compensates the widows of workmen who have been killed in industry. In England the widow receives a sum of money, while in most other countries she receives a pension equal to a part of her husband's earnings. This continues until she remarries, and serves to protect the orphans. In Germany the orphans are thus provided for until their fourteenth year,—the age at which they are allowed to begin earning.

One of the chief aims of the women of Australia, lately organised into a political association in order to concentrate effectively upon social legislation, is to bring about a higher degree of economic security for women who have children to support.

The idea that mothers, who provide citizens for the state, are as fully entitled to state support or pensions during the time when the children need their care as are soldiers, who fight for the state, is gradually making its way as a part of the new ideal.

The subject of industrial compensation may be found in *Workingmen's Insurance*, by William Franklin Willoughby, which is now under revision and is to be published by the Russell Sage Foundation. Of Australian methods Miss Alice Henry, Hull House, Chicago, writes that the united experience of all workers there supports the plan of the maternal subsidy. Its abuse may be readily prevented by careful administration. Though not yet universal, the practice of enabling deserving widows or deserted mothers to keep the home together is spreading in all the States. South Australia gives rations for children if more than one in a family. New South Wales, Western Australia, and Victoria board the children with their mothers to the age of twelve. See *Report* Interstate Conference of Workers among Dependent Children, and *Reports*, State Children's Department, Adelaide, Australia; also *State Children in Australia* by Miss Spence.

APPENDIX E

MINIMUM WAGE BOARDS

"The minimum wage boards were established ... in response to an anti-sweating agitation. ... The social sanction of the minimum wage determinations rests upon the common interest of society in maintaining among all classes of people a standard of living comporting with the general wealth and civilisation of the community, and guaranteeing healthy social progress. ... Minimum wage boards ... are composed of not less than four nor more than ten members representing equally the employers and employees in the trade under their jurisdiction with a chairman elected by the other members but who is not one of the original members of the board. A separate board is formed for each trade."

[*Bulletin of the Bureau of Labour*, vol. x., 1905, pp. 61, 62, Washington.]

"Equal pay for equal work has been partially recognised for the first time in Australia under private enterprise by a recent 'determination' of the Drapery Trade Wages Board. It is already in force in the Federal Public Service, in the Junior Grade of the State Education Department, and now a beginning has been made in private enterprise."

[Vida Goldstein in *Jus Suffragii*, organ of the International Woman Suffrage Alliance, January 15, 1910. Edited by M. G. Kramers, 92 Kruiskade, Rotterdam.]

APPENDIX F

THE LIQUOR TRAFFIC AND ITS ATTITUDE TOWARD WOMAN SUFFRAGE

The National American Woman Suffrage Association prints a leaflet reproducing what it calls a "secret circular" which was distributed by an association of brewers and wholesale liquor dealers in a western State at the time of a campaign to introduce a woman suffrage amendment into the State constitution. This circular came into the possession of the daily press and may be found in newspaper files. It is stated that its authenticity has never been denied. Part of its text runs as follows:

"It will take 50,000 votes to defeat woman suffrage; there are 2000 retailers in ———. That means that every retailer must bring in 25 votes on election day. . . .

"We enclose 25 ballot tickets showing how to vote; we also enclose a postal card addressed to this association. If you will personally take 25 friendly voters to the polls on election day and give each one a ticket showing how to vote, please mail the postal card back to us at once. You need not sign the card. Every card has a number, and we will know who sent it in. Let us all pull together and let us all work. Let us each get 25 votes."

INDEX

A

Abolitionist Congress in Geneva, 77
" " " " resolutions of, 77-79
Accidental infection in syphilis, 31, 38-39
Acquired Syphilis, 10
Age of consent, U. S. laws concerning, 116-121
Ages when girls are ruined, 87-88
Alcoholism in syphilis, 15, 25-27
Antibodies, 10
Anti-serum treatment, gonorrhœa, 48

B

Blindness, in gonorrhœa, 46, 51
Breeding-place of the venereal diseases, 34
Brussels Conference, first, 81
" " resolutions, 83
" " second, 81, 83-89
" " resolutions, 89-90
Butler, Mrs. Josephine E., 69

C

Cancer and syphilis, 24
Chancroid, 52
Clandestine prostitution, 98, 99
Colles, phenomenon named after, 19
Congenital syphilis, 16-17
Constitutional forms of gonorrhœa, 46
Contagious Diseases Acts, The, 68
Continental System of Regulation of Vice, The, 66

Control of prostitution, 59-103
Course of gonorrhœa, 43
Crime and syphilis, 27-29
Crusade of women under Mrs. Butler, 71

D

Dangers of regulation, 93-103
Diplococcus gonorrhœæ, 40
Donné, 5
Double standard of morals, The, 60-62

E

Enfranchisement of women needed, 158-159, 164-166
Extent of prostitution, 152-154

G

Girls, trade in, 108-109
Gonococcus gonorrhœæ, 40
Gonorrhœa, 40
    " and syphilis, 51, 52
    " course of, 43
    " history of, 41-43
    " mortality from, in prostitutes, 50
    " organism of, 40
Great Britain, regulation in, 67-75
Gummata, 16

H

Hard chancre, 12
Heredity, syphilis, 18
History, white slave trade, 104-105
Hours of work, 163

I

Immunity, gonorrhœa, 48
    " syphilis, 20

Index

Incubation period { chancroid, 52
gonorrhœa, 43
syphilis, 11
Infantilism, 17
Initial sore of syphilis, 12
International Federation against vice, formation of, 77

L

Laws covering age of consent in U. S., 116-121
" share of, in white slave trade, 107-108
Legislation, efforts to amend, 109-110, 171 ff
Liquor traffic and woman suffrage, 186-187

M

Martineau, Harriet, warnings by, 68
Mediate contagion, 98
Metchnikoff, Élie, 5
Minimum wage boards, 185-186
Modes of transmission, gonorrhœa, 47-48
"   "   syphilis, 37-39
Moral standard, double, the, 60-62
Morals police, 64
Morbidity of gonorrhœa, 49
"   " syphilis, 29, 31
Mortality from gonorrhœa in prostitutes, 50
Mucous patch, syphilis, 13

N

National Consumers' League, inquiry into wages, 162-163
National Vigilance Leagues, 110-111
Need of knowledge, 133-136
Neisser, experimental work of, 9
"   micrococcus of, 40
"   serum diagnosis of, 9-10
Nervous system and syphilis, 22-24
Numbers of young men infected, 154-155

O

One-child sterility, 45

P

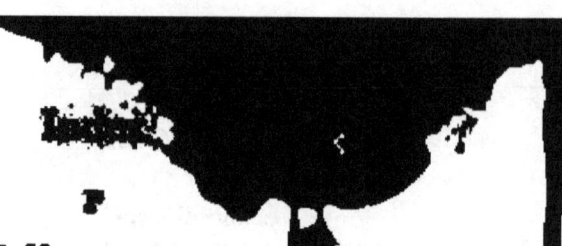

Para-syphilitic diseases, 23
Pasteur Institute, 8
Persevering prostitutes, numbers of, 86
Poverty and prostitution, 156
Prevalence of gonorrhœa, 49
    "   " syphilis, 29
Prevention of venereal diseases, 129-130
   " " " " (individual), 138
   " " " " " childhood, 139-141
   " " " " " youth, 141-142
   " " " " " marriage, 142-145
   " " " " " accidental, 146-149
   " " " " (social) childhood, 150
   " " " " " girlhood, 152
   " " " " " motherhood, 160, 188-9
Primary lesion, syphilis, 12
   " stage " 12
   "   " length of, 12
   " infection in gonorrhœa, 43
Profeta, phenomenon named for, 20
Progress of crusade against venereal disease, 74-75
Prostitutes, mortality of, gonorrhœa, 50
Prostitution, 34-36
   " of minor girls, 86
   " attempts at legislation in U. S., 171
Protest of women against regulated vice, 71
Puberty and syphilis, 17

R

Race suicide, the true, 52
Reasons for prostitution, 155-156
Regulation of prostitution, 59; efforts to secure legislation in U. S., 171
Regulationists in Medical Congress, 1873, 76
Report on Criminal Assault, 176 ff
Resolutions, first Brussels Conference, 83
   " second " " 89-90

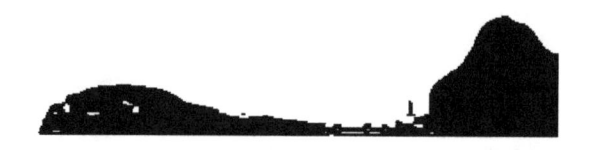

S

Sanitary inefficiency of regulation, 96-99
Schaudinn, discovery, of, 5-6
" organism of, 5
Second stage of gonorrhœa, 44-45
" " " syphilis, 13-14
Select Committee, House of Commons, 75
" " " " Lords on white slave trade, 75
Share of laws, in white slave trade, 107-108
Social legislation needed, 163
Societies, Sanitary and Moral Prophylaxis, 90-91
Soft chancre, 52-53
Source and spread of syphilis, 32
Spirilla refringens, 6
Spirochæte balanitis, 7
" pallida, 5
" " destroyed by heat, 7
" " demonstrated in tissues, 8
Stages of gonorrhœa, 44-45
" " syphilis, primary, 11
" " " secondary, 13
" " " tertiary, 14
Statistics of gonorrhœa, 49-52
" " syphilis, 29-31
Sterility of gonorrhœa, 45-50
Struggle against Contagious Diseases Acts, 73-74
Supreme Court decision, 115
Syphilis, 3,
" acquired, 10
" and carcinoma, 24
" and crime, 27-29
" cause of, 4-5
" alcoholism in, 15, 25-27
" congenital, 10, 16-17
" course of, 10-11
" history of, 4
" mucous patches of, 13
" and the nervous system, 22-24

Syphilis, organism of, 5
" prevalence of, 29
" rash of, 13
" source of, 32
" stages of, 11-14
" statistics of, 29-31
" and tuberculosis, 24-25
" and gonorrhœa, 51, 52

T

Tertiary syphilis, 14
Third stage, gonorrhœa, 46
Three stages, gonorrhœa, 43
Tolerated houses, 65-67
Treponema pallidum, 7
Tuberculosis and syphilis, 24-25

V

Venereal sore, 52-53

W

White slave trade, Europe, 103-104
" " " United States, 110-115
Widowed mothers, protection of, 185, 188-189

Y

Young men infected, numbers of, 154-155

Z

Zeissl, 22

*A Selection from the
Catalogue of*

G. P. PUTNAM'S SONS

**Complete Catalogue sent
on application**

A History of Nursing

The Evolution of the Methods of Care for the Sick from the Earliest Times to the Foundation of the First English and American Training Schools for Nurses.

By LAVINIA L. DOCK, R.N.

Secretary of the American Federation of Nurses and of the International Council of Nurses, etc.

and M. ADELAIDE NUTTING, R.N.

Superintendent of Nurses, The Johns Hopkins Hospital; Principal of Johns Hopkins Training School for Nurses, etc.

Two Vols., 8vo. With 80 Full-Page Illustrations. Net, $5.00

Beginning with the earliest available records of sanitary codes which were built up into health religions, and coming down through the ages wherever the care and rescue of the sick can be traced, through the pagan civilizations, the early Christian works of mercy, the long and glorious history of the religious nursing orders, military nursing orders of the crusades, the secular communities of the later middle ages, and the revival of the deaconess order which culminated in the modern revival under Miss Nightingale, this history is the most serious attempt yet made to collect the scattered records of the care of the sick and bring them all into one unified and sympathetic presentation.

The story is not told in a dry technical fashion, but presents its pictures from the standpoint of general human interest in a subject which has always appealed to the sympathies of men.

Both Miss Nutting and Miss Dock are well known in the nursing world; Miss Nutting, as one of the foremost educators in hospital work, who, as the head of the Johns Hopkins Hospital training school, has so distinguished herself for practical work that she has been called to Columbia University to take the chair of Institutional Management, and her collaborator as a well-known worker for organization and progress, and who, as the secretary of the International Council of Nurses, has already written much on nursing and hospital conditions.

The history is amply illustrated, and contains a copious bibliography of nursing and hospital history.

G. P. PUTNAM'S SONS

New York   London

Books for [...]

A Text-Book for T[raining...]

By P. M. W[ise], M.D., late [...] State Lunacy Commission, etc. [...] by Dr. Edward Cowles, P[hysician...] intendent McLean Hospital.

Second edition. Two volumes, [illustrated...] separately, each . . . .

"This text book has been adopted by the two [State Hospitals?] New York, representing approximately four hundred [pupils?].

Dr. G. Alder Blumer (the medical sup[erintendent of the...] State Hospital) says: "It is an admirable piece of work. [It is] written very clearly, and in language which can be very [easily] understood by the nurse. It covers the whole ground, and [contains] a great deal of matter not to be found in other books, and [with the] adoption of this book other text-books will not be [required for the] training school."

A Text-Book of Materia Medica for Nurses.

Compiled by LAVINIA L. DOCK, graduate of [Bellevue] Training School for Nurses, secretary of the Ame[rican] Federation of Nurses and of the International Co[uncil] of Nurses, etc.

Fourth edition, revised and enlarged. 12°. [...]

"The work is interesting, valuable, and worthy a pos[ition in my] library."—*N. Y. Medical Record.*

"It is written very concisely, and little can be found in it [to criti]cise unfavorably, except the inevitable danger that the stu[dent will] imagine after reading it that the whole subject has been ma[stered.] The subject of therapeutics has been omitted as not a part [of the] nurse's study, and this omission is highly to be commended. [It will] prove a valuable book for the purpose for which it is inten[ded."]—*N. Y. Medical Journal.*

Medical and Surgical Nursing.

A Treatise on Modern Nursing from the Physician's a[nd] Surgeon's Standpoint, for the Guidance of Graduate a[nd] Student Nurses, together with Practical Instruction [in] the Art of Cooking for the Sick. By H. J. O'B[rien,] M.D. 12°. . . . .

G. P. PUTNAM'S SONS, New York and Lond[on]

"*Practical experience speaks from every page of the book—this gives it at once its greatest value and its charm . . . not an idle word—not a shred of padding is to be found between the two covers.*"—*American Journal of Nursing.*

Practical Nursing

A Text-Book for Nurses

By ANNA CAROLINE MAXWELL

Superintendent of the Presbyterian Hospital School of Nursing

—AND—

AMY ELIZABETH POPE

Instructor in the Presbyterian Hospital School of Nursing

Third Edition. Revised. Illustrated. Crown 8vo. $1.75 net. (Postage 12 Cents)

"The appearance of this work, the fruit of the conjoined labors of Miss Maxwell and Miss Pope, marks a turning-point in nursing literature. Up to the present time, the "text-book" and "hand-book" of nursing have treated of subjects which, while they necessarily and indispensably belong in the curriculum of every school for nurses, are yet subjects quite apart from practical nursing in the hospital wards or at the bedside of the sick, and quite out of place in a text-book of nursing. One needs to read the book to appreciate it; a mere enumeration of the subjects gives no hint of the immense amount of care taken to quote methods which have been proved by experience in many schools to be the means best adapted to give good results and at the same time to insure the comfort and confidence of the patient."—*American Journal of Nursing.*

G. P. PUTNAM'S SONS

New York   London

"I consider it the best I have seen and shall recommend its use in our school."—*Kate A. Sanborn, Supt. of Training School for Nurses, St. Vincent's Hospital.*

Essentials of Dietetics
In Health and Disease
A TEXT-BOOK FOR NURSES

By AMY ELIZABETH POPE, Author, with
ANNA CAROLINE MAXWELL
of "Practical Nursing" and Instructor in the Presbyterian Hospital School of Nursing

and

MARY L. CARPENTER
Director of Domestic Science in the Public Schools
Saratoga Springs, N. Y.

Crown 8vo. Illustrated. $1.00 net

Essentials of Dietetics is primarily a text-book, intended to facilitate the teaching of dietetics in schools of nursing. Its aim is to furnish nurses with such information as is indispensable, and can be assimilated in the time given to the study of dietetics in the nursing-school curriculum. It is also adapted to use as a dietary guide for the home. At least one-third of the women who enter the larger schools of nursing do so with the desire of being prepared to take charge of hospitals or to do settlement work, and in both these branches of the nursing profession hardly any one thing is more important than knowing how to direct the buying, preservation, cooking, and serving of food. To do this intelligently it is absolutely necessary to have some knowledge of the chemistry of foods, of the special uses of the various food principles to the body, of the proportions in which they are contained in the different foods, and of the effect on them of acids, heat, salt, digestive ferments, etc.

G. P. PUTNAM'S SONS
NEW YORK   LONDON

"An exceedingly useful and practical book for Nurses"

A Quiz Book of Nursing for Teachers and Students

By

Amy Elizabeth Pope

Joint-Author of "Practical Nursing" and "Essentials of Dietetics"

and

Thirza A. Pope

Together with Chapters on Visiting Nursing

By Margaret A. Bewley, R. N.

Graduate of Presbyterian School of Nursing, and of the Sloane Maternity Hospital, New York City; Instructor in Visiting and District Nursing in Presbyterian Hospital, New York City.

Hospital Planning, Construction, and Equipment

By Bertrand E. Taylor, A. A. I. A.

and

Hospital Book-keeping and Statistics

By Frederic B. Morlok

Chief Clerk in the Presbyterian Hospital, New York City.

Crown 8vo. Illustrated. Uniform with "Practical Nursing."

This book aims to be useful, in the most practical way, to nurses who teach, and to those who are studying under them. It is, in large part, a quiz book, offering in the form of terse question and answer essential information on a wide range of subjects—the information that is essential from the nurse's standpoint. Those who teach will find these questions of assistance when the time they have to devote to preparation for their class work is limited; and those who are taking courses will find the book a great help; especially when studying for examinations.

G. P. PUTNAM'S SONS

New York   London

Second Edition, Revised and Enlarged

Short Talks with Young Mothers

On the Management of Infants and Young Children

By

Charles Gilmore Kerley, M. D.

Professor of Diseases of Children, N. Y. Polyclinic Medical School and Hospital; Attending Physician to the N. Y. Infant Asylum; Assistant Attending Physician to the Babies' Hospital, N. Y.; Consulting Physician, New York Home for Crippled and Destitute Children; Consulting Pediatrist, Greenwich Hospital; Consulting Physician, Savilla Home, N. Y.

Second Edition, Revised and Enlarged
With 21 Illustrations

345 pages, Crown 8vo. $1.00 net. (By mail, $1.10)

Some Critical Comments

"It is full of practical suggestions and has evidently been written by a man who has had wide personal experience in the management of the nursery. It is singularly free from all theoretical bias.

"Every word that Dr. Kerley has to say on the subject of these habits is worth attention and is useful not only for mothers, but for practitioners also, who are frequently consulted on these matters."

"The directions for the feeding of infants and young children are very simple and in accordance with the best modern principles.

"We highly commend the diet schedules which are drawn up for the children of from one year to six years of age."
—*London Lancet.*

"It is one of the books for which persons of experience feel profoundly grateful. . . . This book is clear, sensible, exhaustive, and interesting. It is not too large to be conveniently handled and the print is very clear."—*The Criterion.*

G. P. Putnam's Sons
New York   London

CPSIA information can be obtained
at www.ICGtesting.com
Printed in the USA
LVHW102334021219
639197LV00004B/377/P